Cystitis
UNMASKED

James Malone-Lee MD FRCP

tfm Publishing Limited, Castle Hill Barns, Harley, Shrewsbury, SY5 6LX, UK
Tel: +44 (0)1952 510061; Fax: +44 (0)1952 510192
E-mail: info@tfmpublishing.com; Web site: www.tfmpublishing.com

Editing, design & typesetting: Nikki Bramhill BSc Hons Dip Law
Cover illustration: © 2021 Alex Wilby

First edition: © 2021
Reprinted: January 2021
Paperback ISBN: 978-1-910079-63-8

E-book editions: © 2021
ePub ISBN: 978-1-910079-64-5
Mobi ISBN: 978-1-910079-65-2
Web pdf ISBN: 978-1-910079-66-9

Printed by Gutenberg Press Ltd., Gudja Road, Tarxien, GXQ 2902, Malta
Tel: +356 2398 2201; Fax: +356 2398 2290
E-mail: info@gutenberg.com.mt; Web site: www.gutenberg.com.mt

Contents

Acknowledgements

When we first conceived of this book we considered it being a series of chapters written by the members of our research group, affectionally referred to as "the gang". However, it was eventually decided that I should write the text and that the gang would check my spelling mistakes. This is called delegation; a wise principle of good management.

I chose to write this work in the first-person plural because so much of the content results from the research that these fine people have accomplished during their years of working with our centre. In fact, having completed their postgraduate degrees, the vast majority continue to participate in the research and clinical work of our service.

Thus, I wish to acknowledge the academic contributions of the following successful PhD students of the last 15 years: Rajvinder Khasriya, Anthony Kupelian, Kiren Gill, Harry Horsley, Sanchutha Sathiananthamoorthy, Linda Collins, Jane Currie and Sheela Swamy. In so doing I must thank them for so many happy times and wonderful adventures; then now and to come.

I should also wish to thank my editor, Nikki Bramhill, who thought up the idea for this book and encouraged me to write it. Nikki proved so patient and supportive. When it came to the editorial work her meticulous error-spotting skills evinced a resolution down to 1 pixel — amazing!

I thank my beloved Jenny to whom I have been married for 47 years. Having endured the relentless pressures during the years of censure of our service, she patiently put up with my immersion in this writing. I am most proud of and grateful to Alex Wilby, my son-in-law, whose artistic skills are manifest in these pages.

James Malone-Lee
January 2021

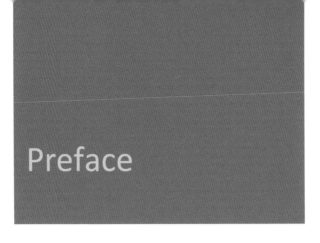

Preface

In November 2019 a 38-year-old woman presented to us seeking advice before her bladder was removed. It was to be the next step in her management. She was being treated with Cystistat® bladder instillations, which despite the pain she had learned to self-administer. She had experienced urethral dilation, cystodistension, and varied antibiotic courses including low-dose prophylaxis. There was a 20-year history of recurrent urinary tract infections, increasing in frequency until she was constantly plagued with painful lower urinary tract symptoms (LUTS). Come August 2020 she had no symptoms and her life had normalised when treated with methenamine and nitrofurantoin without side effects. She still had her bladder. If only this story was exceptional, but it is common in our service. This book is about that problem.

Before you go further please know that this is not a conventional textbook on urinary tract infection (UTI). The heart of this project is the assertion that urine culture, regardless of method, is incompetent at excluding UTI and incapable of identifying a causative organism. A simple claim, eating at a fundamental step in the guidelines and protocols for the management of LUTS. If the gold standard reference for excluding the commonest bacterial infection of mankind is defunct, we have a serious problem.

So, this critique is no unsubstantiated, theoretical opinion or polemic. It is the conclusion from a 30-year experimental series that has tested many alternative hypotheses. The outcomes discredit urine collection, urine dipsticks and cultures. Beliefs about cystitis, interstitial cystitis (IC), and painful bladder syndrome (PBS), or bladder pain syndrome (BPS) have crumbled.

We acknowledge the discord that these findings may cause and so we have repeated salient experiments exhaustively, in different samples and contexts. We accepted the burden of proof and tested the counterarguments, hypotheses and alternative explanations argued to contradict our findings. Despite this detailed scrutiny, our thesis has survived; urinalysis is in a parlous state and the patients are paying a price. We do indeed present evidence to imply that all clinical syndromes, predicated on exclusion of UTI by culture, may be erroneous and the phenotypes should be re-examined. Confidence in the truth of the status quo is no longer credible.

To summarise the scientific thrust of this book we present here a set of conclusions drawn from the available published, peer-reviewed data.

A summary of the facts

The gold standard test for diagnosing urinary tract infection during the last 60 years has been to culture a midstream urine specimen and identify a pure growth of a known urinary pathogen [1].

The threshold counts may be adopted, ranging from 10^2 to 10^6 but these do not escape the facts. The quantitative urinary culture thresholds rest on assumptions that were not properly checked:

- The normal bladder is sterile; it is not sterile — several groups have refuted this [2-9].
- There is a quantitative relationship between the culture results and the probability of infection — culture numbers are more likely to depend on the ease of growth [2, 3, 4, 8-17].
- The infection should be caused by a single species — modern published data imply that mixed organisms is more likely [2, 3, 6, 8, 9, 18].

- Cultures of mixed organisms imply contamination — modern data refute the notion of mixed growth of doubtful significance; they are significant [2, 3, 6, 8, 9, 18].
- If epithelial cells are seen in the midstream urine specimen then it indicates contamination [19] — this is not true; most of these cells come from the bladder and reflect bacterial cystitis [8, 20-26].
- If the culture is negative then there is no infection — this is not true; the cultures are incapable of this property [1, 2, 8-10, 18, 27-32].
- Systemic markers of inflammation such as the ESR and C-reactive protein can exclude a significant infection if negative — this is not true as numerous researchers have found [33-39, 40].

The wrong gold standard

It is common for a patient with appropriate symptoms to be undiagnosed on negative culture. That confuses absence of evidence of disease with evidence of absence of disease. Recently Heytens *et al* have claimed that: "The woman that is visiting you with typical urinary complaints has an infection. There is nothing more to explore". The culture misleads [41]. The influence of guidelines and the imposition of 3-day UTI treatment regimens followed by culture-based treatment seems to be generating a surge in patients with chronic recalcitrant bladder pain and recurrent cystitis who get diagnosed with IC/PBS/BPS.

Treatment failure

Uncertain diagnosis is not alone. The treatment of acute cystitis also has its limitations. RCT data from antibiotic studies have reported microbiological and symptomatic failure in up to 28% and 37% of patients within 4 to 14 weeks of treatment [42]. The treatment of these patients is then directed by discredited cultures.

Conclusion

These are disturbing facts about our practices and the consequences for our patients, thus motivating this work. We wish to explain the science and medicine in an accessible style. We use stories to colour the prose and widen the scope to discuss related factors such as argumentation, data interpretation and evolution, all of which influence our thinking on cystitis. We hope that we have achieved our aims.

Professor James Malone-Lee MD FRCP
Emeritus Professor of Medicine
University College London (UCL), London, UK

References

1. Kass EH. Bacteriuria and the diagnosis of infection in the urinary tract. *Arch Intern Med* 1957; 100: 709-14.

2. Khasriya R, Sathiananthamoorthy S, Ismail S, *et al.* Spectrum of bacterial colonization associated with urothelial cells from patients with chronic lower urinary tract symptoms. *J Clin Microbiol* 2013; 51(7): 2054-62.

3. Wolfe AJ, Toh E, Shibata N, *et al.* Evidence of uncultivated bacteria in the adult female bladder. *J Clin Microbiol* 2012; 50(4): 1376-83.

4. Hilt EE, McKinley K, Pearce MM, *et al.* Urine is not sterile: use of enhanced urine culture techniques to detect resident bacterial flora in the adult female bladder. *J Clin Microbiol* 2014; 52(3): 871-6.

5. Ollberding NJ, Volgyi E, Macaluso M, *et al.* Urinary microbiota associated with preterm birth: results from the Conditions Affecting Neurocognitive Development and Learning in Early Childhood (CANDLE) study. *PloS One* 2016; 11(9): e0162302.

6. Price TK, Dune T, Hilt EE, *et al.* The clinical urine culture: enhanced techniques improve detection of clinically relevant microorganisms. *J Clin Microbiol* 2016; 54(5): 1216-22.

7. Brubaker L, Wolfe AJ. The female urinary microbiota/microbiome: clinical and research implications. *Rambam Maimonides Med J* 2017; 8(2): e0015.

8. Gill K, Kang R, Sathiananthamoorthy S, *et al*. A blinded observational cohort study of the microbiological ecology associated with pyuria and overactive bladder symptoms. *Int Urogynecol J* 2018; 29(10): 1493-500.

9. Sathiananthamoorthy S, Malone-Lee J, Gill K, *et al*. Reassessment of routine midstream culture in diagnosis of urinary tract infection. *J Clin Microbiol* 2019; 57(3): 01452-18.

10. Stamm WE, Counts GW, Running KR, *et al*. Diagnosis of coliform infection in acutely dysuric women. *N Engl J Med* 1982; 307(8): 463-8.

11. Hurlbut TA, 3rd, Littenberg B. The diagnostic accuracy of rapid dipstick tests to predict urinary tract infection. *Am J Clin Pathol* 1991; 96(5): 582-8.

12. Kunin CM, White LV, Hua TH. A reassessment of the importance of "low-count" bacteriuria in young women with acute urinary symptoms. *Ann Intern Med* 1993; 119(6): 454-60.

13. Gorelick MH, Shaw KN. Screening tests for urinary tract infection in children: a meta-analysis. *Pediatrics* 1999; 104(5): e54.

14. Deville WL, Yzermans JC, van Duijn NP, *et al*. The urine dipstick test useful to rule out infections. A meta-analysis of the accuracy. *BMC Urol* 2004; 4: 4.

15. Khasriya R, Khan S, Lunawat R, *et al*. The inadequacy of urinary dipstick and microscopy as surrogate markers of urinary tract infection in urological outpatients with lower urinary tract symptoms without acute frequency and dysuria. *J Urol* 2010; 183(5): 1843-7.

16. Walsh CA, Siddins A, Parkin K, *et al*. Prevalence of "low-count" bacteriuria in female urinary incontinence versus continent female controls: a cross-sectional study. *Int Urogynecol J* 2011; 22(10): 1267-72.

17. Kupelian AS, Horsley H, Khasriya R, *et al*. Discrediting microscopic pyuria and leucocyte esterase as diagnostic surrogates for infection in patients with lower urinary tract symptoms: results from a clinical and laboratory evaluation. *BJU Int* 2013; 112(2): 231-8.

18. Bartlett RC, Treiber N. Clinical significance of mixed bacterial cultures of urine. *Am J Clin Pathol* 1984; 82(3): 319-22.

19. Collier S, Matjiu F, Jones G, *et al*. A prospective study comparing contamination rates between a novel mid-stream urine collection device (Peezy) and a standard method in renal patients. *J Clin Pathol* 2014; 67(2): 139-42.

20. Dalal E, Medalia O, Harari O, Aronson M. Moderate stress protects female mice against bacterial infection of the bladder by eliciting uroepithelial shedding. *Infect Immun* 1994; 62(12): 5505-10.

21. Rosen DA, Hooton TM, Stamm WE, *et al*. Detection of intracellular bacterial communities in human urinary tract infection. *PLoS Med* 2007; 4(12): e329.

22. Smith YC, Rasmussen SB, *et al*. Hemolysin of uropathogenic *Escherichia coli* evokes extensive shedding of the uroepithelium and hemorrhage in bladder tissue within the first 24 hours after intraurethral inoculation of mice. *Infect Immun* 2008; 76(7): 2978-90.

23. Thumbikat P, Berry RE, Zhou G, *et al*. Bacteria-induced uroplakin signaling mediates bladder response to infection. *PLoS Pathog* 2009; 5(5): e1000415.

24. Hannan TJ, Mysorekar IU, Hung CS, *et al*. Early severe inflammatory responses to uropathogenic *E. coli* predispose to chronic and recurrent urinary tract infection. *PLoS Pathog* 2010; 6(8): e1001042.

25. Horsley H, Malone-Lee J, Holland D, *et al*. *Enterococcus faecalis* subverts and invades the host urothelium in patients with chronic urinary tract infection. *PloS One* 2013; 8(12): e83637.

26. Collins L, Sathiananthamoorthy S, Rohn J, Malone-Lee J. A revalidation and critique of assumptions about urinary sample collection methods, specimen quality and contamination. *Int Urogynecol J* 2020; 31(6): 1255-62.

27. Latham RH, Wong ES, Larson A, *et al*. Laboratory diagnosis of urinary tract infection in ambulatory women. *JAMA* 1985; 254(23): 3333-6.

28. Hooton TM. Practice guidelines for urinary tract infection in the era of managed care. *Int J Antimicrob Agents* 1999; 11(3-4): 241-5.

29. Naber KG, Bergman B, Bishop MC, *et al*. EAU guidelines for the management of urinary and male genital tract infections. Urinary Tract Infection (UTI) Working Group of the Health Care Office (HCO) of the European Association of Urology (EAU). *Eur Urol* 2001; 40(5): 576-88.

30. Epp A, Larochelle A, Lovatsis D, *et al*. Recurrent urinary tract infection. *J Obstet Gynaecol Can* 2010; 32(11): 1082-101.

31. Gupta K, Hooton TM, Naber KG, *et al*. International clinical practice guidelines for the treatment of acute uncomplicated cystitis and pyelonephritis in women: a 2010 update by the Infectious Diseases Society of America and the European Society for Microbiology and Infectious Diseases. *Clin Infect Dis* 2011; 52(5): e103-20.

32. NICE. Urinary tract infection (lower) — women. London: National Institute for Health and Care Excellence, 2014. Available from: http://cks.nice.org.uk/urinary-tract-infection-lower-women#!topicsummary.

33. Garin EH, Olavarria F, Araya C, *et al*. Diagnostic significance of clinical and laboratory findings to localize site of urinary infection. *Pediatr Nephrol* 2007; 22(7): 1002-6.

34. Kotoula A, Gardikis S, Tsalkidis A, *et al*. Comparative efficacies of procalcitonin and conventional inflammatory markers for prediction of renal parenchymal inflammation in pediatric first urinary tract infection. *Urology* 2009; 73(4): 782-6.

35. Ayazi P, Mahyar A, Daneshi MM, *et al.* Diagnostic accuracy of the quantitative C-reactive protein, erythrocyte sedimentation rate and white blood cell count in urinary tract infections among infants and children. *Malays J Med Sci* 2013; 20(5): 40-6.

36. Feldman M, Aziz B, Kang GN, *et al.* C-reactive protein and erythrocyte sedimentation rate discordance: frequency and causes in adults. *Transl Res* 2013; 161(1): 37-43.

37. Xu RY, Liu HW, Liu JL, Dong JH. Procalcitonin and C-reactive protein in urinary tract infection diagnosis. *BMC Urol* 2014; 14: 45.

38. Koufadaki AM, Karavanaki KA, Soldatou A, *et al.* Clinical and laboratory indices of severe renal lesions in children with febrile urinary tract infection. *Acta Paediatr* 2014; 103(9): e404-9.

39. Julian-Jimenez A, Gutierrez-Martin P, Lizcano-Lizcano A, *et al.* Usefulness of procalcitonin and C-reactive protein for predicting bacteremia in urinary tract infections in the emergency department. *Actas Urol Esp* 2015; 39(8): 502-10.

40. Shaikh N, Borrell JL, Evron J, Leeflang MM. Procalcitonin, C-reactive protein, and erythrocyte sedimentation rate for the diagnosis of acute pyelonephritis in children. *Cochrane Database Syst Rev* 2015; 1: CD009185.

41. Heytens S, De Sutter A, Coorevits L, *et al.* Women with symptoms of a urinary tract infection but a negative urine culture: PCR-based quantification of *Escherichia coli* suggests infection in most cases. *Clin Microbiol Infect* 2017; 23(9): 647-52.

42. Milo G, Katchman EA, Paul M, *et al.* Duration of antibacterial treatment for uncomplicated urinary tract infection in women. *Cochrane Database Syst Rev* 2005; 2: CD004682.

Dedication

I am dedicating this book to the many

people — women, men and children

whose lives have been wrecked by the

horrors of the disease that I write about.

I do so hope that one day, for them:

"All shall be well, and all shall be well,

and all manner of thing shall be well."

Julian of Norwich (1342-1416)

Chapter 1

The intriguing history of urinary tract infection

The history of medicine is full of cautionary tales relevant to modern practice, but we keep reoffending, returning enthusiastically to the mistakes of the past. Why should this be? Perhaps this story of cystitis may shed some light on this bizarre mystery.

Cystitis is one of our most common bacterial diseases. It is much assumed to be a simple, uncomplicated condition which resolves easily. In 70% of cases that is true, but when unchecked it proves itself an appalling affliction, devastating lives and wreaking untold misery. Regrettably, the 30% who prove unresponsive are frequently the victims of intolerance. Science tells us how to respond to the 30% but modern guidelines, which just address the 70%, insist on rejecting what science suggests. There is worse to come since the ill-considered use of 'big data' threatens to average exceptional patients out of consideration.

Sumerian clay tablets from Mesopotamia (3000 BCE), Babylonian tablets (1700 BCE), and Egyptian hieratic writing in the Ebers Papyrus of circa 1500 BCE describe uroscopy, the contemplative examination of the urine. These civilisations recognised three groups of healers: physicians, priests and sorcerers. For urinary tract infection (UTI), the Egyptians prescribed rest and herbs, prayers, incantations and spells, and hence the necessity for a multidisciplinary team. As this book develops we shall see that we do not appear to have advanced much on that.

Prayer remained an important intervention for many centuries. The Greeks invoked Asklepios in seeking health, but it is unknown whether there was a god for UTI. However, come Christianity and the Middle Ages, the hermit St. Vitalis of Assisi (1295 to 1370) became the patron saint of bladder and genital afflictions. Should you consider a pilgrimage, his relics are preserved at San Vitale, a small village near Assisi in Italy, where today our patients gather to pray for deliverance from the torment that has defied our protocols; there's a huge problem with crowd-control.

A secular approach to health care came with the Greeks, notably Hippocrates (460 to 377 BCE). The Hippocratics rejected prayers, spells and potions insisting on natural responses to disease: promoting rest, nutrition, healthy lifestyles and herbal supplements. The Hippocratic oath is a laudable declaration, albeit including some trade-guild protectionism. One sentence, "I will not use the knife, not even, verily, on sufferers from stone, but I will give place to such as are craftsmen therein", fosters the separation of physicians from surgeons; a principle most relevant to this tale. The axiom "First do no harm" is not Hippocratic; it derives from a phrase used by Auguste Chomel (1788-1858), a Parisian pathologist, but we raise it here because it is important, if misattributed.

In *The Aphorisms* [1], the Hippocratics (there were more authors than Hippocrates) wrote 19 axioms on urine and they are shrewdly perceptive. "If a patient passes blood, pus, and scales, in the urine, and if it has a heavy smell, ulceration of the bladder is indicated" is a good evocation of cystitis and "When bubbles settle on the surface of the urine, they indicate disease of the kidneys, and that the complaint will be protracted" may describe the surface tension effects of proteinuria, a hallmark of nephritis, not UTI. These Greeks recognised the antiseptic properties of urine which they applied to burns and other skin lesions. Urine does indeed contain numerous antimicrobial substances, which we sabotage through dilution by recommending increased fluid intake when treating cystitis.

It was the Hippocratics, borrowing from the Sumerians and Babylonians, who fashioned the theory of the four humors: black bile, yellow bile, phlegm, and blood, with disease being attributed to an imbalance in these. The associated temperaments occur in common parlance; melancholic, choleric, phlegmatic and sanguine. These reflect our obsession with categories, which, as we shall see, is folly because biological systems abhor categorisation. Humorism came to dominate medical thinking, largely unchallenged, for the next 2000 years. Humoral thinking was adaptable, persuasive, mouldable to different circumstances and self-validating. Similarly today, plausible explanations, lacking empirical evidence, abound in medicine, so that imaginative invention, wrapped in jargon, is often used to answer inconvenient questions.

The medical superstar of the classical world was Galen; the Greek physician to the households of the emperors Marcus Aurelius, Commodus and Severus. He was a graduate of Pergamon and Alexandria, and a Hippocratic. Galen was a deeply studious man who had absorbed all of Greek medicine, including humorism. He was a disciplined anatomist, a teacher, prolific writer and a brilliantly effective surgeon. He understood the importance of cleanliness, sterility and disinfection, as well as the holistic Hippocratic principles of rest and nutrition. He emphasised the causes of disease over their effects. In a classical physiological experiment Galen demonstrated that urine was manufactured by the kidney. We should pity the poor primate that provided the evidence.

Galen's achievements were extraordinary and his influence dominated the Middle Ages and Renaissance. Regrettably, he was too prolific for the transcribers of his writing so they penned abstractions that omitted many of his intellectual reflections. This precious, classical wisdom journeyed from the Greek scripts to Arabic texts of the Mediterranean Muslim culture, to Latin written in translation schools, particularly in Spain. This knowledge was modified through a scribal, transcription chain influenced by local opinion. These abstracts formed the core of university medieval medical education from the twelfth to the sixteenth century. Ultimately, the sophisticated scientific analyses of the Hippocratics and Galen were reduced to didactic recipes, foreshadowing modern-day guidelines.

From the fifth century, much health care was provided by the monastic hospitals. Hippocratic principles of cleanliness, rest and nutrition were combined with humorism through blood-letting and herbs. It might be hoped that a 1000 years of trial and error, with monastic knowledge exchanged through monastic networks, might have evolved a herbal grail, buried in some ancient library. The selection pressure was not very specific since the monks understood herbs to provide general humoral treatment, as was the view in folk practice. David Allen and Gabrielle Hatfield [2] spent 16 years documenting the herbal folk remedies of the British Isles and ■ Table 1.1 describes their relevant data for the urinary tract. The vernacular names evoke magical powers; sadly, this is not to be.

Table 1.1. Herbal remedies for the urinary tract [2].

Linnaean taxonomy	Vernacular name
Urinary complaints	
Agrimonia eupatoria	Agrimony
Arctium spp.	Burdock
Arctostaphylos uva-ursi	Bearberry
Elytrigia repens	Common couch
Euphorbia spp.	Spurge
Linum catharticum	Fairy flax
Malvaceae	Mallow
Persicaria bistorta	Bistort
Pilosella officinarum	Mouse-ear hawkweed
Ruscus aculeatus	Butcher's broom
Stellaria media	Chickweed
Vaccinium myrtillus	Bilberry
Veronica beccabunga	Brooklime
Cystitis	
Achillea millefolium	Yarrow

During the sixth century, Theophilus Protospatharius published a treatise *De Urinis*, which introduced the medieval world to Greek views on uroscopy (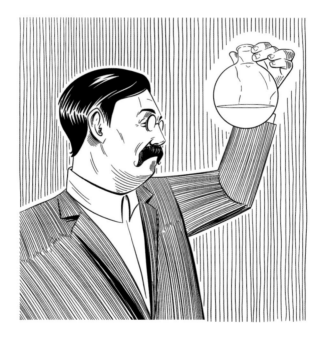 Figure 1.1). Theophilus described a complex chromatic scale for thick and thin urine. He provided instructions on how to interpret appearances. *De Urinis* was a popular work being a source of pseudo sagacious knowledge for impressing clients. The matula, a bladder-shaped glass vessel specific to uroscopy, was a badge of expertise. Come the Renaissance, physicians were diagnosing by uroscopy alone, without taking a history or examining the patient as may happen today with a dipstick test or culture. Uroscopy provided lucrative opportunities for charlatans, some inventing uromancy for divination. Eventually, in 1637, Thomas Brian published *Pisse Prophet* which

Figure 1.1. Uroscopy fabricates the illusion of percipience — the sagacious physician contemplates the qualities of the urine and in applying his esoteric learning, discerns what is ailing the patient. Is this so different today when we dipstick and culture the urine? *Illustration courtesy of Alex Wilby.*

exposed this nonsense. Sadly, there were plenty of phonies ready to move in to replace uroscopy. Today, tests abound, few properly verified, and in later chapters we shall have long-overdue confrontations with urinalysis, urodynamics and cystoscopy. Beware! An investigation can be invented and used to define a disease, detectable only by the same investigation — it is a meaningless, self-validating imposter with urodynamics being an excellent example.

At the beginning of the eighteenth century, Antonie Philips van Leeuwenhoek, a Dutch draper and scientist, ground his own lenses to produce an effective, simple, single-lens microscope which he used to discover "animalcules", which we understand to be microbes. The early compound microscopes, with two or more lenses, whilst increasing magnification, suffered from spherical and chromatic aberration caused by greater diffraction of light at a lens periphery and refractive differences caused by wavelength. In short they were not much good. It took until the mid-nineteenth century before aberration was tamed. Today, the available scientific evidence implies that the compound microscope is the most important instrument that we have for the management of cystitis; nothing else has been able to compete. So why is microscopy not taught in some medical schools? Why should it be excluded from nursing curricula?

During the nineteenth century, Paris became the hub of clinical methods, the meticulous history and examination dominating medical practice. French medicine had a profound influence on the Canadian physician, William Osler, the "Father of Modern Medicine", who coined the truism: "Just listen to your patient, he is telling you the diagnosis". How often is a patient with lower urinary tract symptoms exposed to tests before, or in place of, a history and examination?

It was the Germans who developed laboratory medicine at this time. Thus, Karl Weigert first stained bacteria in 1875. Robert Koch isolated and cultured the first bacillus in 1876. Theodor Escherich discovered *Escherichia coli* in 1885. In 1881, Fanny Hesse developed the use of agar-based culture. Her husband, Walther Hesse, working with Koch, used the agar method in the discovery of the tubercle bacillus but they never acknowledged Fanny. Does that sound familiar? The failure of senior academics to attribute correctly and to claim for themselves the achievements of their subordinates causes so much harm to all of us.

Ignaz Semmelweis (1818-1865) used statistical analysis of outcomes to discover that puerperal fever could be transmitted from a corpse, an infected vagina and/or an infected ulcer to mothers in labour, on the practitioner's hands. He found that this could be prevented by hand washes with carbolic (phenol) prior to touching patients. This history has become fictionalised because of the allure of the monomyth [3]: the romantic, outcast, pilgrim-hero, ultimately vindicated is a recurring medical fable that is nowadays a bit of a cliché. It is heartening that colleagues were supportive of Semmelweis, despite his difficult personality. His findings did spread through Europe, particularly in the UK, because his colleagues promoted his ideas. Unable to cope with criticism, Semmelweis refused to present his findings and delayed writing them up, eventually penning a rambling, indigestible book. He suffered from bipolar depressive disease and eventually developed organic brain disease which caused him to be admitted to an asylum. There he died from sepsis caused by a finger infection. The monomythical story of the profession closing ranks is appealing but not so true. The historian Roy Porter [4] observed that Semmelweis was up against the widely accepted miasmatic theory, another plausible, adaptable and attractive story.

Louis Pasteur (1822-1895) was a master of experimental science and a microscopist to his core. He validated the germ theory of disease and refuted the doctrine of spontaneous generation. Robert Koch (1843-1910) discovered the microbes responsible for tuberculosis, cholera and anthrax, proving the case for infectious disease. He published *Koch's Postulates* (see ▓ Table 1.2 overleaf) which proposed how to prove microbial causation from culture data. These postulates have exerted an unfortunate influence on our understanding of urinary infection, so we shall return to them.

Table 1.2. *Koch's Postulates* **for establishing a microbe as a cause of a disease.**

1	The organism must always be present, in every case of the disease.
2	The organism must be isolated from a host containing the disease and grown in pure culture.
3	Samples of the organism taken from pure culture must cause the same disease when inoculated into a healthy, susceptible animal in the laboratory.
4	The organism must be isolated from the inoculated animal and must be identified as the same original organism first isolated from the originally diseased host.

On 24 November 1859, Charles Darwin published *On the Origin of Species by Means of Natural Selection, or the Preservation of Favoured Races in the Struggle for Life* [5]. This was described by Daniel Dennett as "The single best idea anybody ever had" [6]. In 1868, RB McKenzie whilst criticising Darwin provided a perfect summary, here paraphrased: "The intricate creations of nature occurred despite the absolute ignorance of the artificer". All that evolution requires is random variation, replication, selection pressures and time [7]. It is a process of trial and error elimination.

Darwinian evolution is important, fulfilling a crucial explanatory role in the story of cystitis. It may surprise you that we shall invoke it often in the pages of this book. Evolutionary mechanisms can be adapted to developments in human thought and scientific discovery. In fact scientific evolutionary epistemology [8, 9] is the most successful discovery method in human history, which inexplicably, the evidence-based medicine movement excludes.

The correction of lens aberration in the compound microscope enabled Hottinger [10] in 1893 to measure the excretion rate of white blood cells in urine. Nevertheless, the technique is usually attributed to Addis (1925) [11]. The method was laborious and impractical but improvements were achieved and by the 1960s pyuria counts were established so that the finding of ≥ 10 wbc/mm^3, of unstained, unspun urine examined in a haemocytometer, was considered a diagnostic threshold of UTI. Unfortunately, the reference depended on mistaken assumptions about urine culture.

In 1896, Sigmund Freud described "psychoanalysis"; a method that licenses conjecture to explain symptoms. It was justified on the sagacity of the analyst and the privileged knowledge he possessed. It self-validates because, in the therapist's opinion, the analysis explains the case impeccably. If you dissent, that is because of your psychological maladjustment generating resistance and not a scientific viewpoint. This grotesque humbug has sired medicine's great god of the gaps; psychosomatics. It is ingenious; if a patient does not get better, the clinician can blame her by invoking a psychological aetiology. Frewen (1978) opined "The unstable bladder of functional origin is a frequent psychosomatic disorder". "Functional" was a synonym for psychosomatic and a pseudo diagnosis.

At the end of the nineteenth century, the medical literature described the use of organic acids to treat UTI: benzoic acid, biboric acid (boric acid) and others. Hippuric acid was first synthesised by a French chemist in 1853. It was a Russian who synthesised hexamethylenetetramine which was introduced as a urinary antiseptic in 1899. As methenamine mandelate, it became the leading treatment for UTI during the first half of the twentieth century. Recently, as methenamine hippurate, we have brought it from retirement to star in the show.

During the nineteenth century, observations of preferential staining of bacteria initiated an exploration of coal-tar derivatives for stains with antibacterial properties. After a lengthy process of "trial and error elimination" (evolutionary epistemology), Gerhard Domagk discovered that a red dye, produced by Bayer, worked, saving his daughter from amputation. Thus, Prontosil, a prodrug, initiated the age of antibiotics. It was developed by Bayer who were also responsible for aspirin. But let us pause for some history: during the Third Reich Bayer was part of IG Farben which manufactured Zyklon B, a powerful cyanide-based pesticide. SS-Obersturmbannführer Rudolf Höss, the commandant of Auschwitz, claimed to have murdered over 2,500,000 people with Zyklon B. Fritz ter Meer supervised the slave-labour operations of the IG Farben plant at Auschwitz. After the war he became president of Bayer. We should never forget this.

Prontosil was rapidly superseded by the Pasteur Institute's discovery that the simpler, cheaper and more effective para-aminobenzenesulfonamide could be manufactured from the prodrug. Nevertheless, Gerhard Domagk received his Nobel Prize in 1945.

The cephalosporins were discovered in 1948 from Sardinian sewerage effluent. Ampicillin semisynthetic derivatives of penicillin, and the first aminopenicillin, came out in 1961, with amoxicillin following in 1972 and amoxicillin/clavulanic acid (co-amoxiclav, Augmentin) in 1984. The urinary disinfectant, nitrofurantoin, was developed in 1953. Nalidixic acid came out in 1962 and was subsequently developed into the quinolones. Cefalexin was developed in 1967. The 1970s saw the emergence of pivmecillinam from Finland, trimethoprim/sulfamethoxazole (TMP/SMX; co-trimoxazole) an American invention and fosfomycin (phosphonomycin) a Spanish discovery of 1969, found in soil.

Since 1957, the diagnosis of urinary tract infection (UTI) from culture of a mid-stream urinary specimen (MSU) has rested on criteria described by Kass (1957) [12]. He reported that MSUs from 25 patients with chills, fever, flank pain and dysuria had grown more than 10^6 bacteria colony forming units per ml (cfu/ml). After studying the MSU in asymptomatic people, he concluded, "For survey purposes, a count of 10^5 bacteria or more per ml of urine has been designated arbitrarily as the dividing line between true bacilluria and contamination". Bacteria that "were not generally considered to be pathogens of the urinary tract" were excluded in favour of "common pathogens of the urinary tract" so that the Kass criterion was qualified with the phrase "known urinary pathogen". Kass never claimed to define a diagnostic threshold for UTI, but we adopted 10^5 cfu/ml as that demarcation between UTI/no UTI with calamitous consequences. The problem illustrates the folly of presumption. We assumed that the normal bladder was sterile and that Koch was right in insisting on a single causative organism. Borrowing from Jane Austen [13]: "What we conjectured one minute, we believed the next"; it is not a wise tendency.

This book will explore the situation today and develop these themes. We shall learn that the lessons of the past have had limited influence on the practices of today. We shall see just how badly the guidelines, protocols and accepted wisdom have fared. This story is further coloured by recent dogmatic imposition of mistaken practice which has caused such dreadful suffering. Medicine has probably always had its surfeit of people who, convinced of their own rectitude, bustle the world righting the wrongs of their colleagues. They leave Emma Woodhouse straggling. Perhaps they thrive in the contemporary faddish obsession with central planning, its rules, processes, procedures and penalties. But this lacks an insightful grasp of the extreme complexity of human biology, an inevitable consequence of the mechanisms of Darwinian evolution, which thrives on contingency. There never were standard solutions and we define best practice at our peril. Random variance, exceptions, unpredictability and multiplicity defy the doctrinaire, as has always been the case. Instead of regulations, we should be better served by the scientific outlook and methods developed to function under uncertainty [14, 15]. It is not subversive or obstreperous to ask that we rediscover the skilful practice of medicine based on the clinical history and examination because the necessary competence starts there [16].

References

1. Pormann PE. *The Cambridge companion to Hippocrates.* Cambridge, UK; New York: Cambridge University Press; 2018.

2. Allen DE, Hatfield G. *Medicinal plants in folk tradition: an ethnobotany of Britain & Ireland.* Portland, Or; Cambridge: Timber; 2004.

3. Campbell J. *The hero with a thousand faces*. New York: Pantheon books; 1949.

4. Porter R. Hospitals and surgery. In: Porter R, Ed. *The Cambridge history of medicine*. Cambridge: Cambridge University Press; 2006: 199.

5. Darwin C. *On the origin of species by means of natural selection, or the preservation of favoured races in the struggle for life*. London: John Murray; 1859.

6. Dennett DC. *Darwin's dangerous idea: evolution and the meanings of life*. London: Penguin; 1996.

7. Dennett D. Darwin's "strange inversion of reasoning". *Proc Natl Acad Sci USA* 2009; 106 Suppl 1: 10061-5.

8. Gontier N. Evolutionary epistemology as a scientific method: a new look upon the units and levels of evolution debate. *Theory Biosci* 2010; 129(2-3): 167-82.

9. Popper KR. *Objective knowledge: an evolutionary approach*. Revised ed (reprinted with corrections and a new appendix 2). Oxford: Clarendon Press; 1979.

10. Hottinger R. Uber quantitative eiterbestimmungen im harne nebst. Bemerkungen uber centrifugiren und sedimentiren. *Zbl Med Wiss* 1893; 31: 255-6.

11. Addis T. The number of formed elements in the urinary sediment of normal individuals. *J Clin Invest* 1925; 2: 409-12.

12. Kass EH. Bacteriuria and the diagnosis of infections of the urinary tract; with observations on the use of methionine as a urinary antiseptic. *AMA Arch Intern Med* 1957; 100(5): 709-14.

13. Austen JA. *Sense and sensibility: a novel*. London: T. Egerton; 1811.

14. Taleb N. *Antifragile: how to live in a world we don't understand*. London: Allen Lane; 2012.

15. Taleb NN. *The black swan: the impact of the highly improbable*, 1st ed. London: Allen Lane, Penguin; 2007: 366.

16. Mazur DJ. A history of evidence in medical decisions: from the diagnostic sign to Bayesian inference. *Med Decis Making* 2012; 32(2): 227-31.

Chapter 2

Evidence fair, fake and fashionable

We wish to address the principles of scientific proof and probability early in this book because UTI has been plagued by data interpretation errors that have been the cause of much confusion and misery for patients. We hope to present the case in a manner that is readily understood by the average clinician who may have no formal training in statistics and probability. Whilst we must discuss some statistical principles, we are going to do so using plain language without equations and with liberal use of graphs. It is not necessary to command great statistical knowledge to understand and our intention is to equip the reader with enough to ask important questions when peddled nonsense by enthusiasts. This knowledge should prove valuable for wider application outside of UTI.

Let us revisit the eighteenth-century Enlightenment and the empirical scientific method which has achieved so much for humanity (Figure 2.1). The traditional clinical method is an exercise in this process [1, 2]. We start by collecting data from a history and examination as taught by William Osler [3]. These data* are assimilated through induction. Abduction formulates a hypothesis, or hypotheses; a differential diagnosis is a good example. Deduction generates a prediction that must be true if the hypothesis is true. We then test for the occurrence of the prediction. If the prediction is falsified, the hypothesis is rejected by error elimination and the cycle is repeated. A test is only valid if it is applied in this manner. The data assimilated from the history and examination are all important and their relevance may not be

---

*   Datum is singular; data are plural.

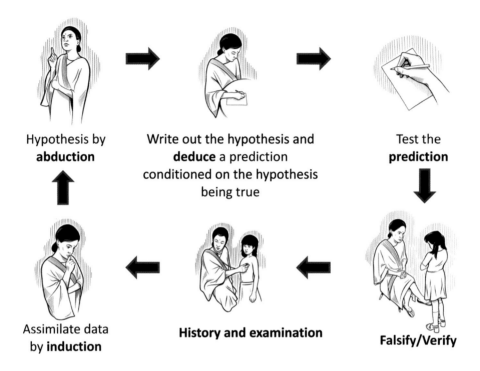

Hypothesis by abduction

Write out the hypothesis and deduce a prediction conditioned on the hypothesis being true

Test the prediction

Assimilate data by **induction**

History and examination

Falsify/Verify

Figure 2.1. The empirical scientific method applied to the clinical assessment. *Illustration courtesy of Alex Wilby.*

We shall return to this circuit over and again in this book and illustrate it in a variety of different forms. It is so important. The key in this image is pace, reflection and being circumspect about the use of tests. In the developing world, tests are far less available and the doctors depend heavily on their clinical skills. We should argue that they may well practice better medicine than in the developed western world.

dismissed on the results of a test. It is a common error to predicate the patient's symptoms and signs, giving precedence to the test result; this is a path to the gates of doom.

The folly of dichotomisation

We shall start by addressing tests, because doctors are voracious consumers. Beware, tests are not the champions that they are built up to seem. They have the capacity for much mischief.

Many think that tests provide reliable, binary outcomes; "positive" or "negative". They never achieve this because there are additionally, false positives and false negatives, which are commonplace. ▨ Figure 2.2 tables the four outcomes from any test with a binomial result. Later, we shall use this table to explore some inconvenient facts about probability, the first being that a randomly selected person, from the general population, testing positive is more probably showing a false positive than a true positive. Because we crave security, abhorring risk, we refuse to countenance this

	The true state	
	Positive	Negative
Test result — **Positive**	True positive	False positive
Negative	False negative	True negative

Figure 2.2. The four potential outcomes from a dichotomised test.

likelihood; "What if I miss something?" Thus, gratuitous testing and screening wreak havoc, because abundant false positives provoke additional investigations to reassure the patient and clinician. Wilkins Micawber is a character in Dickens's 1850 novel *David Copperfield*; a comical optimist given to claiming, "Something will turn up". Much testing reflects Micawber's ideology and it is a barren nonsense.

False negatives create similar mayhem, especially when the test is insensitive. Patients present to clinics with symptoms and signs typical of urinary tract infection. At the reception their urine is tested by dipstick and/or culture which prove negative. The patients are incorrectly told that they do not have a UTI. If a history and examination had been achieved, the high prior probability of a UTI would swamp the test data. A false negative test obtained before the consultation encourages anchoring bias, where we fix on the first piece of information given, so that the clinician is primed to make a mistake by dismissing the symptoms and signs.

The siren call to venerate a test as the ultimate arbiter is seductive because it shields us from the worries of intellectual engagement; the test accepts all blame. However, the truth is that any result that contradicts expectations raised by the history and examination is probably false and doubting the test result is not an opportunistic contrivance but a commitment to the rules of probability. Conflicting results mandate reconsideration of all data, not a fawning deference to the test. What is the purpose of a history and examination when their assimilation is dismissed on a test outcome? This wacky recommendation abounds in the algorithms found in our guidelines [4].

What would you say if we insisted that a rainbow is either violet or red and nothing else? It makes little sense and so it is with the "positive"/"negative" categorisation of the diagnosis of UTI; it is a false dichotomy. In 2011, Richard Dawkins published an essay in the *New Statesman* entitled "The tyranny of the discontinuous mind", which drew on a chapter in *The Ancestor's Tale* [5]. The article provides a lucid dissection of the errors caused by categorisation; it pays reading. Immanuel Kant insisted that categories, whilst useful devices of the imagination, had no existence in reality [6]. Darwin never tired of emphasising the gradualism of evolution [7]. Nevertheless, our organisations strive to enforce categories on medical practice.

Examine ▓ Figure 2.3, which provides an abstract image of the spectrum of UTI, from no disease to terminal sepsis — there are no demarcations; it is folly to categorise continua. In ▓ Figure 2.3, we indicate a demarcation that reflects the Kass criterion of $\geq 10^5$ cfu/ml; an arbitrary boundary between UTI and no UTI; this is no different to insisting that a rainbow is red or violet; a Procrustean mutilation of a biological system. The pervasive influence of dichotomisation is reflected in the popularisation of ROC curve analyses** in the clinical literature. These methods are not appropriate to biological

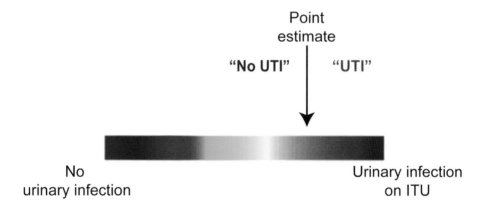

Point
estimate

"No UTI" | "UTI"

No
urinary infection

Urinary infection
on ITU

Figure 2.3. A biological continuum applied to urinary culture results associated with UTI.

These data align along a continuum spanned between no UTI and very serious life-threatening infection. The use of an arbitrary border between "No UTI" and "UTI" is vandalism and provoking of serious trouble.

** Receiver operating characteristic (ROC) curve developed in World War II to analyse radar signals not urinalysis.

variables; they are inimical to the properties of continua, so ignore them — they are bad for your patients and for you.

Do not ignore the base rate

It is necessary to explain some terminology: sensitivity, specificity and predictive values. This will be much like a stroll across a minefield, but we shall help you to pull yourself together at the end.

Figure 2.4 is a derivative of Figure 2.2. We assess a binary test result against a reference. There should always be a reference standard because tests can only provide relative values. Later, we shall discuss tests, used in urinary tract medicine, having no reference, which is truly bizarre. The variables "true positive", "false positive", "false negative" and "true negative" are counts. The following derived variables are commonly used: sensitivity, specificity, positive predictive value and negative predictive value. When someone says "derived", reach for your parachute, it may get messy.

		The reference standard	
		Positive	Negative
Test result	**Positive**	True positive count	False positive count **Type 1 error**
	Negative	False negative count **Type 2 error**	True negative count

Figure 2.4. The nomenclature of a binomial test.

A type 1 error is a false positive result when the patient is healthy. A type 2 error is the false negative result when the patient is sick.

The **sensitivity** of a test is the proportion of persons, **with the condition**, who are detected by the test:

$$\text{Sensitivity} = \frac{\text{True positive count}}{\text{True positive count} + \text{False negative count}}$$
(The sum count of those **with** the disease)

The **specificity** of a test is the proportion of persons, **without the condition**, who test negative:

$$\text{Specificity} = \frac{\text{True negative count}}{\text{True negative count} + \text{False positive count}}$$
(The sum count of those **without** the disease)

The sensitivity and specificity are worked out on a specific sample of patients who are **known** to have, or not to have, the condition. When we test in the clinical context, our patient may not match that sample. We shall have to make allowance for that.

Before we go further, there are two other derived values that should be addressed to warn you off because they are exceedingly misleading and should be ignored, despite the enthusiasm with which they are bandied around.

The positive predictive value is the proportion of all positive results that were correctly positive **in the sample studied**.

$$\text{Positive predictive value} = \frac{\text{True positive count}}{\text{True positive count} + \text{False positive count}}$$
(The sum of all **positive** tests)

The positive predictive value is falsely synonymised with the probability that a patient has the disease, given a positive test.

The negative predictive value is the proportion of all negatives, **in the sample studied**, that were correctly negative.

Negative predictive value = $$\frac{\text{True negative count}}{\text{True negative count} + \text{False negative count}}$$

(The sum of all **negative** tests)

These predictive values are limited strictly to the sample that was studied. We should not extrapolate to the general population or worse, to the individual case. You will read papers on test validation blithely reporting the predictive values without acknowledging their serious limitations.

If you visit Wikipedia, you will discover many other derived variables related to test results. Some doctors learn these in order to impress colleagues at the grand round. In truth, they are very crazy things which are best ignored; they would perturb your equanimity.

The positive and negative predictive values are seductive because they impersonate the probability of the disease, given a positive test and conversely the probability of no disease, given a negative test. They do not, but we shall now explain how to work out those probabilities correctly.

We speak of the probability (P) of an event (A) and write this as "P(A)". We also speak of an event (A) GIVEN an event (B) and write this as "P(A|B)" which means P(A **GIVEN** B); "|" means "GIVEN". We capitalise GIVEN because it is so important. Always question: "Given what?" when discussing diagnoses and test results.

Human cognition is not well adapted to probability theory and we struggle to grasp it. The equations can be tricky to follow, and the concepts are not intuitive. It would be inappropriate for us to describe the derivation of the relevant equations here. However, we can provide a most useful rule of thumb.

The probability of disease, given a positive test, is proportional to the sensitivity multiplied by the prevalence of the disease:

*The probability of **disease** if test **positive** ∝ sensitivity × prevalence*

The converse, in relation to a negative test is:

*The probability of **no disease** if test **negative** ∝ specificity × (1 − prevalence)*

Note that we substituted in "test negative", "specificity" and "1 − prevalence"; the latter, because the proportion with disease, plus the proportion without disease, must add up to 1 so the proportion without disease must equal 1 − prevalence.

The key variable to focus on is the prevalence, as it applies to the patient in front of you, which sires this question: "Before I do this test what is the probability that this person has a UTI given the history, symptoms and signs?" This is the best estimate of the probability of disease before the test was accomplished. A test rarely has the capacity to refute that prior estimate and certainly not the UTI tests.

When you reflect on that question, please understand that the prevalence is NOT the prevalence in the nation, but the prevalence in the subpopulation that best fits the patient that you are treating. We have been repetitious because so much relevant literature appears to confuse population prevalence with the probabilities applicable to the individual. The imprudence of extrapolating generalisations from notably specific observations crops up often in this book.

A negative urinalysis is more likely a **false negative** in a patient with a typical history, symptoms and signs than in someone with none of these. The prevalence is much higher in those with a history, symptoms and signs; (1 − prevalence) is commensurately smaller, which lowers the probability of no disease, given a negative test.

So, it is a gaffe to dismiss the UTI diagnosis, for a symptomatic patient, given a negative test. The test data must be interpreted in light of the history and examination of the patient of interest. We are duty bound, to correct the test result for other factors that were gleaned from this clinical assessment. If you are beginning to wonder why we do tests you are on the right path.

Suppose that the specificity of a test is 95% or 0.95 and the prevalence of a UTI in 80-year-old female diabetics with appropriate symptoms is 95%, then the probability that a negative test, from such a person, is a **true negative** $\propto$ 0.95 x (1 − 0.95) = 0.05 = 5%. This may come as a bit of a shock. Tragically, such a patient will very likely be told that she could not have a UTI. Some will assert their certitude by stating that the specificity is 0.95 and so claim that "the diagnosis is 95% certain". This is a very bad situation.

The error caused by not considering the relevant prevalence is the formal logical fallacy of "ignoring the base rate" which means the same as ignoring the prior or ignoring the prevalence. Human cognition influences our assimilation of data so when presented with complicated information, gleaned from the clinical history (base rate information), followed by specific figures such as data from a test, our minds are prone to exclude the former and focus solely on the latter. Exactly this error is promoted in numerous guidelines and is widespread in clinical practice. Dipstick tests done at the surgery door, without consideration of a history and examination, are similarly fallacious. Arguing that you do not have time, compounds the aberration with the logical fallacy of "special pleading"; exempting yourself from the rules of logic by claiming special dispensation.

The Bayesian equation that governs this analysis is as follows:

$$\text{The probability of disease if test positive} = \frac{\text{Sensitivity x Prevalence}}{\text{Probability of a positive test}}$$

The probability of disease if a test is positive is called the "**posterior probability**".
The prevalence is called the "**prior probability**".
The sensitivity is called the "**likelihood**".
The probability of a positive test is called the "**marginal probability**".

Posterior probability = $$\text{Posterior probability} = \frac{\text{Likelihood} \times \text{Prior probability}}{\text{Marginal probability}}$$

The marginal is the probability of a positive test whether true or false. It is a normalising function that ensures the posterior probability calculates as a fraction. It is not that important; it is tricky to follow, and we advise you not to worry about it. Thus, we excluded it from our rule of thumb above.

Beware! There are some profound persons who will strut and fret about the veracity of the prior probability. In practice, it is not a significant worry. It is an estimate, improved by a careful history and examination. We apply Bayes' theorem through chains of calculations with the posterior probability of one calculation being the prior probability the next, so the accuracy improves with each observation in the sequence. When computing such chains in artificial intelligence (AI) we start with a "universal prior" which is neutral.

Bayesian inference [8] provides a more appropriate approach to understanding clinical data; it includes the base rate data and rejects the black and white frequentist approach that generates "p" values and dichotomised "Yes/No" answers. It is nuanced, and sensitive to the complex, multi-faceted nature of human life experience. It is not necessary to understand the Bayesian equations in order to grasp the principles. It is possible to get by with a basic appreciation of the influence of the contributory factors.

The rules of probability force us back onto the clinical history and examination. Tests have a seductive appeal in a world of expediency with productivity-driven protocols. A test creates an illusion; a quick, efficient answer, when we must hurry. It is a fallacy, with deplorable consequences.

Excluding the exceptions

We must now address another reckless tendency which is the habit of extrapolating from the general to the particular.

Figure 2.5 plots a frequency distribution of the log pyuria counts (wbc/µl) obtained from 1217 of our patients at their first attendance. This is a large sample number and deliberately so. First and foremost, this distribution is positively skewed with a long tail. Taking the log of data is a means of reducing the skew of the distribution. In this case it did not work because the skew is too great. Such distributions are notably common in clinical practice, a troublesome fact rarely admitted. The long tail represents exceptions and outliers that are inconvenient to those seeking a tidy set of statistics, as when planning or directing health care provision. We were cautioned about this in Nassim Taleb's bestseller, *The Black Swan* [9].

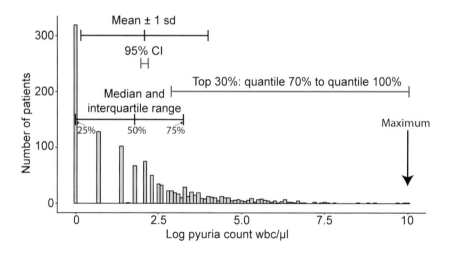

Figure 2.5. Frequency distribution of log pyuria count at first attendance. CI = confidence interval; sd = standard deviation.

Many clinical distributions are skewed like this. The popular myth is that the normal distribution is the most common and this is not true. Skewed distributions are normal amongst patients.

To emphasise the contrast, in ▓ Figure 2.6 we provide a similar plot of a 3000-patient normal distribution, simulated by the statistical programming language "R", which we love deeply although we must admit to increasing episodes of infidelity with the Johnny-come-lately Python.

The purple bar-line plots the mean with one standard deviation either side. For normally distributed data (▓ Figure 2.6) this is a reasonable assessment of the dispersion. When the data are from a continuum, as in ▓ Figure 2.3, they are described as **parametric data**; hence **parametric statistics**. The brown line describes the median and interquartile range, which is advised for non-

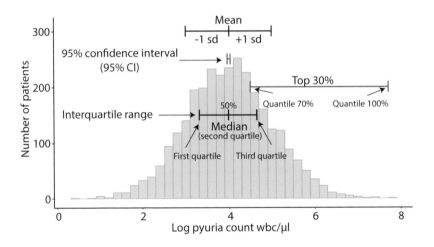

Figure 2.6. Frequency distribution of log pyuria from a normal distribution. CI = confidence interval; sd = standard deviation.

Even when a population is normally distributed there will still be outliers which should not be removed from consideration. If a distribution is truly random normal, then repeated sampling is bound to pull out an exception, as occurs too often with gratuitous testing.

normal distributions and discontinuous data, when they are described as **non-parametric**; giving us **non-parametric statistics**. The interquartile range does a bad job at summarising the skewed data of ▓ Figure 2.5. Just because a method is recommended it does not necessarily achieve its purpose.

The blue bars define the 95% confidence interval, which is an important construct. There is no need to understand how this is calculated but appreciating its meaning is invaluable. If we take samples repeatedly from this patient population and calculate the mean of each of the samples, 95% of the sample means will lie between these bounds of the 95% confidence interval, even if the samples are not normally distributed.

Thus, if we obtain a sample "X", calculate the mean and find that it does not lie between the bounds of the interval, we can be 95% confident that our sample "X" comes from a different population to that represented by the 95% CI. We can write "p<.05". This is the whole basis of the "p" value. We have illustrated this in ▓ Figure 2.7 where we have loyally used the statistical software "R" to simulate some results from three different experiments. In each case we compare two sampled groups; red and blue. We have plotted the resulting means and 95% CI with the relevant p-values underneath. It can be seen how the positions of the means relative to the 95% CI of the comparator governs the p-value.

This is a good point to add a caution. Many tests are promoted on statistically significant differences between groups as plotted in ▓ Figure 2.7. Some claim that patient/control group differences from enhanced quantitative urine culture (EQUC) and 16S rRNA urine genomics implies the ability to identify the offending microbe. This is a fallacy because differences are not the same as causation. Judea Pearl describes the three rungs of the ladder of causation [10]:

- Correlation.
- Intervention.
- Counterfactual.

We shall get to this later; for now, we should explain that between group differences are the same as correlation. Most know the slogan that correlation is not the same as causation.

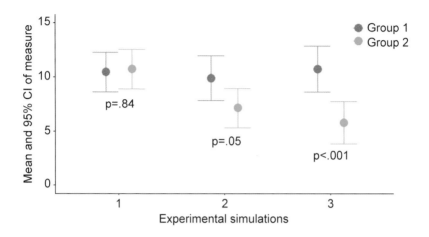

Figure 2.7. The mean and 95% CI from three different experiments comparing two sampled groups.

The ability to generate a significant p-value of p<.05 hinges on the position of the mean of Group 1, shown in red in the boundaries of the 95% confidence interval of Group 2, shown in blue. If the means are not overlapped by the comparator 95% CI, then the p-value must be less than .05 and the groups differ statistically significantly. There is nothing to be gained by chasing lower values because the p-value is no measure of effect size. The 95% CI gives you so much more information than the p-value in isolation.

Figure 2.7 describes differences **and** correlations; the mathematics of analysis of variance (ANOVA), which measure differences, and the general linear model (GLM) regression/correlation are the same. It is just that ANOVA was developed in biological sciences and GLM in the social sciences; they are not different. Correlation is only the first rung of the ladder of causation. For a microbial isolation test to be valid it must detect the causative microbe(s). Figure 2.7 does not achieve that. Those who promote EQUC such as broth cultures and 16S rRNA next-generation sequencing (NGS) molecular methods ignore that.

Confusing correlation as causation is a powerful, infectious meme; the essence of all advertising used fanatically by salesmen. We cling to the message as if our lives depended on it. It is still false despite our heartfelt wishing. Culture and NGS do not identify cause; but so many pay for them.

In the examples of ▦ Figures 2.5 and 2.6, the 95% CI interval is very narrow. This is because the sample size is so large (1217). The larger the sample size, the narrower the 95% CI. This property opens the 95% CI to manipulation by using excessively large samples so as to achieve a significant p-value and thereby dupe everyone when an effect size is pathetic. This is a common subterfuge invariably camouflaged by complicated statistical verbigeration. Tell it to your bewildered patients, "This nostrum will work wonders; it doesn't do much but it has great p-values".

The most important annotation in ▦ Figure 2.5 is the red line which bounds 30% of observations, forming the long tail of inevitable exceptions [9]. The long tail recurs over and again in medicine. Because 30% of the data points lie along the tail of exceptional events, the probability of any of many rare exceptional events is 30%, and these are not covered in our protocols. That is almost 1 in 3. The use of summary statistics, whether parametric or non-parametric, results in exclusion of these patients from consideration in many clinical trials, guidelines and diagnostic thresholds. This error haunts UTI and has wrought harm.

The meta-analyses of randomised controlled trials (RCTs) on antibiotic treatment of acute UTI show that 3-day and 14-day antibiotic courses fail between 25% and 35% of patients. Unfortunately, you must dig through the data tables to spot the existence of these exceptions which are lost in the summary statistics. Tests for UTI are deficient because their validations ignore skews. It is silly to summarise these data with point estimates such as means or medians. As illustrated in ▦ Figure 2.3, it also makes no sense to have diagnostic threshold points based on summary statistics; they are not going to work. "Interstitial cystitis" was invented out of the ether to explain away the effects of a long tail and it has failed calamitously.

There is an important principle touched on in ▦ Figure 2.5: 315 patients (26%) had no pyuria at presentation. When we analysed data collected at subsequent assessments, only 102 (8%) failed to show pyuria. A one-off test does not necessarily capture all the salient data and, as was the case here, a negative test measured when the clinical history, symptoms and signs point to a high prevalence is far more likely to be a false negative than a true negative. As an historical note, we managed the 26% on their symptoms and signs and that got us into some trouble. Were we right or wrong? The answer is expressed as a probability distribution.

It is sometimes argued that large samples and meta-analysis are adopted to include a broad span of the population of interest thereby increasing the probability that the findings will be applicable to the specific patient in your clinic. This is a laudable aim, but the summary statistics subvert this by averaging out the exceptions.

Many find long tails, outliers and exceptions irksome and inconvenient to the legitimacy of extrapolations, based on "the average patient", which are referenced in health strategies, guidelines and algorithms. These patients are not accommodated by an ordinary consultation; they require more time and tend to have more than one problem. The long tail describes random events, which are impossible to predict [9]. How do you commission services and clinical governance for patients who exhibit unanticipated disease variations? It is very annoying of them, so it is not surprising that we have found ways of "disappearing" exceptions from our consideration. One way is to ignore them, camouflaging them in complex data reports [11]. Another option is to use the central limit theorem.

Figure 2.8 is a plot of 100,000 data elements sampled from a simulation generated by the "R" programming language; it is a skewed distribution much like the pyuria data we showed earlier. The tail of this distribution is not convenient. So, we can handle this by collecting samples (trials) from the population, calculating the mean of the samples (trial mean) and then calculating the mean of the means (grand mean). What a great way of summarising the results of several trials. They do this in meta-analyses so it must be a splendid idea. The central limit theorem states that the distribution of the means of means (grand mean) will approach a normal distribution as the number of means entering the calculation rises, even if the population is skewed; hallelujah!

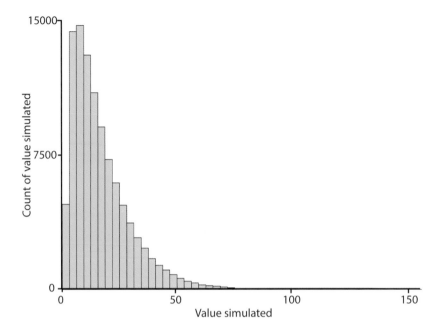

Figure 2.8. Frequency distribution from a positively skewed simulation.

A skewed population like this is called positively skewed because the tail is in a positive direction. This skew was not responsive to log transformation but we shall see in Figure 2.9 that repeated sampling with a grand mean of sample means had no trouble in achieving a normal distribution.

    Figure 2.9 shows the results of applying the central limit theorem, broken up into stages, where a series of simulations are plotted out. Sample one, described in the top panel, plots the frequencies of 300 numbers drawn from the same skewed distribution used to generate   Figure 2.8. We call this process a trial. The top panel is an ordinary frequency distribution of a sample; unlike the subsequent panels it is not a distribution of means of samples.

    In the second panel, we act differently by doing five trials each of 300 numbers. We calculate the individual means of each trial, giving us five means and then we calculate the mean of those five means to give us one mean of means, or a grand mean. We repeat the process 300 times to achieve 300 grand means which are plotted out in a frequency distribution.

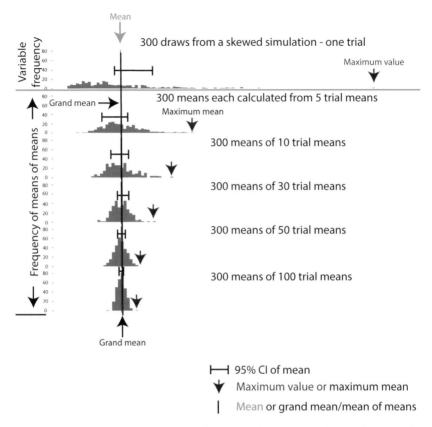

Figure 2.9. Demonstrating the effect of the central limit theorem in removing exceptions.

There are two factors at play in this illustration. First, the size of the samples and then the use of means of means. At first glance the grand mean of all the sample means seems a sensible summary statistic but given the complex heterogeneity of human pathophysiology this method overlooks much that is important.

As we move down through the panels the number of trials that are run increases through 10, 30, 50, 100 numbers, but the method similarly calculates the means of the means of the trial means, repeating 300 times to achieve 300 means of means for the plot.

We have drawn the 95% confidence interval bars spanning the vertical line that marks out the mean of the top panel and the grand mean of the lower

31

panels; regardless, the mean is always the same. The red short arrows are important because they indicate the maximum value plotted. The reduction in the maximum demonstrates how outliers can be removed from consideration, or to use contemporary vernacular, cancelled.

These panels illustrate several important properties:

- The 95% CI narrows in the second and subsequent panels, and is narrower compared to the top panel. This is a key effect of using means of means. Thus, less of the distribution is acknowledged.
- The 95% CI narrows with increasing the sample size; n=10; 30; 50; and 100. This property is co-opted when large samples are used to increase the probability of a desired p-value when the effect size is small.
- The red arrows flag the maximum values, which stand proxy for the exceptions. These creep in closer to the mean of means with increasing numbers of trials. Thus, we can remove the exceptions from consideration by using means of means and increasing the sample sizes.

The disappearing exceptions may occur in meta-analyses and the effects have come to haunt our understanding of the treatment of UTI. Guidelines are developed based on "1a" grade evidence that imply patients will behave similarly to a theoretically average patient that may be unrealistic [4, 11]. The effect can be limited by summarising only raw, disaggregated data that are not summarised. Nevertheless, large samples still have the potential to mislead, so we should suspect them.

Feedback loops

This is not some pretentious exercise in data theory for enthusiasts. The aftermath of our temporary clinic closure in 2015 was peppered with various reviews and investigations. As we worked through this, it dawned on us that our scrutineers did not grasp the scale of the chronic UTI (cUTI) problem. Some appeared baffled by the patients. A few seemed to believe that a tiny minority of educated, middle class, vociferous women were creating a storm in a teacup. They may have been articulate and stroppy but that does not invalidate the truth in their message.

We answered to assessors who, whilst lacking experience of the core patients, were well versed in policy, process, procedure and the numerous guidelines. Perhaps this was symptomatic of the growing bureaucratisation of our health care systems; a flight from reality fed by procedural abstractions. What stood out was the polar contrast in the attitudes of the local councillors and many members of parliament (MPs), from all sides who involved themselves. In their case, a hackneyed word, empathy, is truly appropriate; it was so impressive.

There is an interesting movement in prison reform that is showing great promise. It addresses the fact that offenders rarely have contact with the victims of their crimes and do not understand the many effects of their actions. The restorative justice movement brings perpetrators and victims together to explore the consequences of the offender's misdeed [12]. Similarly, our built-in clinical service feedback systems force us to face the consequences of what we do, particularly when we fail, and it is not always congenial. It may be beneficial if those who formulate patient management policies, which they feel compelled to impose on their clinical colleagues, did have to meet with the patients who are adversely affected by their decisions or were apprised of the adverse outcomes. Clinicians serving the various committees will claim such patient feedback. However, the 2020 Independent Medicines and Medical Devices Safety Review report by Baroness Cumberlege, which we shall cover in Chapter 3, vehemently contradicts that. If we separate authority from authentic responsibility, the consequences are frequently regrettable.

Regression to the mean

Daniel Kahneman learned the influence of this phenomenon when working with Israeli fighter pilots [13]. Berating pilots for performing badly on tasks was associated with ensuing improvement. However, if good performance was praised it was followed by deterioration. This led to a belief in scolding without positive feedback. It was the blighted pilots who forced Kahneman to spot the error. The pilot performances were caused by regression to the mean; regression effects. Function below your mean one day and you will probably perform better next time and vice versa. Your performance randomly oscillates about a mean. Decisions based on sparse data risk similar error. Accuracy requires distributions from several measurements. It is unwise to treat on point estimates and better to think graphically, attending to trends. A further subversion of regression effects occurs when a test is repeated until the desired result is achieved and that desired point outcome is used in isolation.

Regression effects explain most of the claims made for quack remedies and the misattribution of placebo effects. In the wider world, many actions, like sacking football managers, selling falling shares, rebuking juniors, similarly fail to understand random oscillations and regression effects.

Imagine that you are an external advisor, or similar meddler [14]. You are appointed to attend to an underperforming organisation. Random variation is your best friend. You arrive during a trough performance; things get better because of regression effects; all you must do is bullshit and pocket the pay cheque. The phenomenon is the essence of those bragging, "Didn't we done a doddle" yarns — "Na it's in ya regressions mate, innit". Always return to check if the triumph was sustained.

It is appropriate for executives to use summary statistics and aggregate data. However, an officious leadership may misjudge by censuring individual performance without recognising the randomness of the distributions that inform their synopses.

The antidote heuristic is always to use a graph and we shall return to this later, illustrating with a graph.

The tyranny of the p-value and dodgy artifices

Our troubles are further aggravated by the insistence on dichotomising the complex human data collected during clinical trials; so that a continuum is beaten into binomial categories: "the treatment works" ($p \leq .05$)*** versus

---

*** The form $p<.05$ is correct and not $p<0.05$ because p will never exceed 1 so the zero is superfluous.

"the treatment doesn't work" (p>.05). The odds ratios much favoured in meta-analysis are similarly limiting but we are told that the quality of such evidence is Grade 1a. How can this be?

This leads us to the analysis of clinical trial data and the use of p-values to decide whether the findings are significant or not significant. The p-value answers this about the data: "If there were no real effect, what would be the probability of an effect size equal to or greater to that measured by this experiment?" If you think about it, this is not informative.

This brings us back to the all-important effect size which we should explain in some detail. Let's say we run an experiment consisting of two similar samples of patients taken from the same population. We treat one sample "P" with a placebo and the other "A" with a medication. We measure one outcome variable at the start (P_0 & A_0) and 6 weeks later (P_6 and A_6). It is a fact of life that both samples will change during the period of treatment whatever they are taking. We calculate this change:

Change on placebo = $P_6 - P_0 = P_{change}$

Change on active treatment = $A_6 - A_0 = A_{change}$.

The effect size is the difference in these changes.

Effect size = $A_{change} - P_{change}$

The effect size can be written as the 95% confidence interval of the between group difference in change; an excellent, honest declaration. It is not well recognised that this interval renders the p-value nigh on redundant; if the interval does not span zero the result is statistically significant (p<.05); we need not know more. If the p-value were let go, the quack industry would require bereavement counselling.

$A_{change} - P_{change}$, the between group difference, is the most important measure, because it tells us something about the effect of treatment. A p-value provides no such information. The quack remedies and some dubious treatments are promoted by advertising A_{change}, the within group difference, which is so disingenuous. The same error is committed when people defend their outcomes by claiming that the condition is subject to a placebo effect. We shall return to this when we discuss treatment.

The mathematics dictates that no matter how small an effect size, and ineffective a treatment, given enough numbers of subjects, the desired p-value is always achievable. Thus, a large clinical trial can make much of a pathetic effect size by boasting a significant p-value.

Figure 2.10 plots the results of two simulations generating normally distributed data. The graphs illustrate the proportion of patients scoring on an outcome whose values are distributed along the axis. One population has

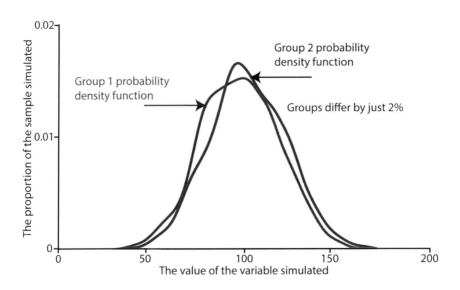

Figure 2.10. Probability density function for two normal distributions differing by 2%.

It would be so much more informative if the between group data were plotted in this way. The Bayesian statistical analysis will always report with a probability density function such as this.

an average score of 100 with the maximum in the sample being 162. The other population has an average score of 102 with a sample maximum of 172. These two groups differ by the trivial amount of 2% which is of no material value.

We have used these simulated data to run some comparative trials of the outcome scores achieved in a sequence of experiments with increasing sample sizes and the results are plotted in Figure 2.11.

We have marked the statistically significant differences with a "*", which emulates a thoroughly bad habit, and written the p-value and the sample size beneath. It can be seen how large sample sizes increase the probability

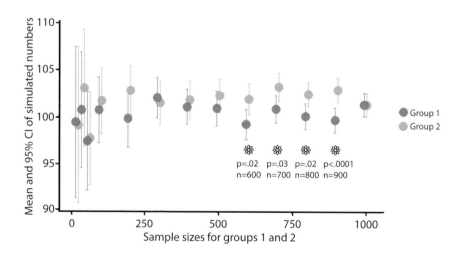

Figure 2.11. The mean and 95% CI of a measure simulated in two groups that differ by just 2%. The plots demonstrate the effects of sample size on statistical significance.

There is no clinically significant difference between the two groups; it is only 2%, but the large samples overcome that inconvenience and it is possible to dupe many people by going on about the p-value which is <.0001 with the n=900.

of a significant p-value despite the difference between the groups being trivial. ▦ Figure 2.11 illustrates another aberration. If you look at the origin of the y-axis it is set at 90; it should be zero. This is the technique of suppressing zero on the y-axis to create the illusion of a greater effect than the reality. ▦ Figure 2.12 corrects this manipulation, sets the y-axis origin at zero and brings the p-value nonsense down to earth.

▦ Figure 2.12 injects some reality into the situation. The suppression of the y-axis zero is a common artifice and you should stay alert to this.

It might be surmised that if a significant difference can be found with small samples, then the effect size would be likely to be more impressive. This is

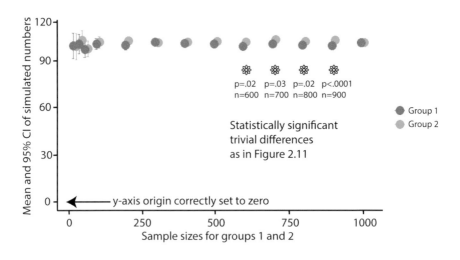

Figure 2.12. The mean and 95% CI of a measure simulated in two groups that differ by just 2%; as in Figure 2.11 but without suppression of the zero on the y-axis.

Using the correct zero for the origin for the y-axis gets the significant differences into perspective. The between group differences are pathetic but the high samples still achieve the coveted p-value.

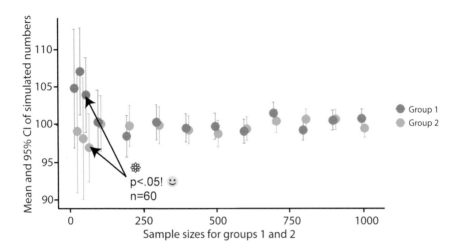

Figure 2.13. The mean and 95% CI of a measure simulated in two groups that differ by just 0.5% to demonstrate how random chance can produce a statistically significant result with low sample numbers. We can increase the probability of such occurrences by measuring multiple outcome variables.

A lucky break using a small sample size. This, we should put down to random chance and not a true effect. It took a significant number of different simulations to get this with a sample of 60 in each group. Had we used multiple outcome measures it would have been a walk in the park. Outcome multiplicity is another way of conning us.

true, but only if this occurs over several repeated experiments. Be alert to statistical opportunism. Figure 2.13 plots a chance occurrence, using the same data, but this time with a 0.5% difference between groups. We rejected a significant number of simulations before we got these results. However, if we had used more than one outcome measure, we should have found this convenient result much quicker. Always consider what has not been reported.

The sample numbers that we used in these simulations are not exaggerations. The digoxin studies in heart failure exemplify huge sampling; in one recent case the sample size was over 21,000 subjects [15], which raises the suspicion that the digoxin effect size may be small. A study of solifenacin [16] recruited 1281 patients when comparing its efficacy against tolterodine and placebo. We used a 20-patient placebo-controlled, crossover study to demonstrate the efficacy of botulinum toxin injections into the bladder [17]; there was a large effect size and our study reported correctly.

There is a difference in the perspective of the partnership between patient and clinician compared to the statistician, epidemiologist and corporate executive. They are equally legitimate but unalike. It is not foolish or obstructive for practising clinicians to insist that their understanding be respected; it is a duty of care. Their perceptions might be irksome and unwelcome, but kindly listen. A practising clinician may relate a truth, disbelieved by others because data summaries have clouded the facts. Governance might favour abstractions for deriving rules, but this is medicine responding to the complex, contingent morass of biological variance. It is naïve to pretend that it can be encapsulated in a set of common threads. We need variability of practice to catalyse the evolution of knowledge.

Silly vernacular

There is the vexed matter of jargon. What does an odds ratio tell you about the effect size? Not much — "there was a statically significant difference". Oh really, what does that tell you about patient benefit? "We rejected the null hypothesis at the 95% level of confidence". What on earth does that orotund expression mean to the average mortal? It is even more baffling because the null hypothesis refers to the opposite of the question you were trying to answer. This weird, pretentious language is needlessly opaque and useful only for covering up inconvenient truths.

What do we need to know?

- What was the difference in the change in outcome measure on active treatment, compared to the same change on placebo?

- Was that difference in change enough to be useful clinically?
- How confident are you in this result?

Let us all cease talking nonsense and describe our purpose, actions and experimental findings in plain language for all to understand.

Solutions

The frequentist comparison of the difference between groups, or the difference in change effected by various interventions or placebo, are important methods provided that they are reported appropriately. The 95% confidence interval of the difference, or the difference in change are the seminal summary statistics which should be stated up front, presiding over all of the other statistics.

Medicine should be a discipline of science, and clinical practice should be based on understanding the pathophysiology of the relevant disease. Scientific evidence should inform our patient care and this knowledge should be treated with respect. The regulatory bureaucratic habit of restricting evidence to RCT data and meta-analyses is not a thoughtful approach to science which strives to consider ALL the data. The argument that time and resources mandate expedient practices is special pleading; if you cannot do it properly then do not do it. Guideline committees are perverse in their insistence on forcing their estimate of "best practice". We have an addiction to binomial "yes/no" decision boxes and a habit for averaging away the exceptions. How is it that meta-analyses are crowned Grade 1a evidence? Where is the critical analysis of the assumptions that justify this? As we shall see, when it comes to UTI treatment, meta-analyses have bungled it badly [11], whilst non-RCT science has discovered answers [18]. The health economists crave predictable standardisation to feed their models; who said biology was predictably exception-free [9, 19]? Ill-informed, autocratic clinical governance, obsessed with rules, imposes practices with punitive glee and deplorable consequences for the patients [20]. These fads and fashions do harm, and, in this book, we explain how in this small field of UTI the damage has been severe indeed.

It is variation, with trial and error elimination, that is the essence of clinical scientific discovery [21, 22]. Scientific evolutionary epistemology [23] inspired by the Enlightenment has been the most successful discovery method in human history [24]. We are smothering it because of an addiction to tidy rule making. Innovation does not flow from imposed top-down planning.

Let us return to William Osler's comment, "Just listen to your patient, he is telling you the diagnosis" [25], because that is where we are going to start. We shall remain loyal to that principle in the coming pages. We know that in this chapter we have attacked many popular assumptions without describing to you our reader, viable alternatives. We shall do that with care and diligence in the coming pages.

References

1. Locke J, Yolton JW. *An essay concerning human understanding.* London: Dent; 1993.

2. Popper KR. *Conjectures and refutations: the growth of scientific knowledge.* London: Routledge; 2002.

3. Castillo-Torres SA, Estrada-Bellmann IE, Lees AJ. Sir William Osler's 'influences' for the successful physician, a reappraisal after 126 years. *Arch Med Res* 2018; 49(6): 418-20.

4. Anger J, Lee U, Ackerman AL, *et al.* Recurrent uncomplicated urinary tract infections in women: AUA/CUA/SUFU guideline. *J Urol* 2019; 202(2): 282-9.

5. Dawkins R. Amphibians — the salamander's tale. In: Dawkins R. *The ancestor's tale: a pilgrimage to the dawn of life.* London: Weidenfield & Nicholoson; 2004: 252-62.

6. Kant I. Transcendental doctrine of the elements. In: Meiklejohn JMD, Ed. *The critique of pure reason.* Penn State Electronic Classics, 1st ed. Philadelphia: The Pennsylvania State University; 1885: 49-74.

7. Darwin C. *On the origin of species by means of natural selection, or the preservation of favoured races in the struggle for life.* London: John Murray; 1859.

8. McGrayne SB. *The theory that would not die: how Bayes' rule cracked the enigma code, hunted down Russian submarines, & emerged triumphant from two centuries of controversy.* New Haven Conn: Yale University Press; 2011: xiii, 320.

9. Taleb NN. *The black swan: the impact of the highly improbable,* 1st ed. London: Allen Lane, Penguin; 2007: 366.

10. Pearl J, Mackenzie D. *The book of why: the new science of cause and effect.* London: Allen Lane; 2018.

11. Milo G, Katchman EA, Paul M, *et al.* Duration of antibacterial treatment for uncomplicated urinary tract infection in women. *Cochrane Database Syst Rev* 2005; 2: CD004682.

12. Shapland J. Forgiveness and restorative justice: is it necessary? Is it helpful? *Oxford Journal of Law and Religion* 2016; 5(1): 94-112.

13. Kahneman D. *Thinking fast and slow.* London: Penguin Books; 2012.

14. Grove AS. *High output management,* 2nd ed. New York: Vintage; 1995.

15. Eisen A, Ruff CT, Braunwald E, *et al.* Digoxin use and subsequent clinical outcomes in patients with atrial fibrillation with or without heart failure in the ENGAGE AF-TIMI 48 trial. *J Am Heart Assoc* 2017; 6(7): e006035.

16. Chapple CR, Rechberger T, Al-Shukri S, *et al.* Randomized, double-blind placebo- and tolterodine-controlled trial of the once-daily antimuscarinic agent solifenacin in patients with symptomatic overactive bladder. *BJU Int* 2004; 93(3): 303-10.

17. Ghei M, Maraj BH, Miller R, *et al.* Effects of botulinum toxin B on refractory detrusor overactivity: a randomized, double-blind, placebo controlled, crossover trial. *J Urology* 2005; 174(5): 1873-7.

18. Swamy S, Barcella W, De Iorio M, *et al.* Recalcitrant chronic bladder pain and recurrent cystitis but negative urinalysis: what should we do? *Int Urogynecol J* 2018; 29(7): 1035-43.

19. Taleb NN. *Fooled by randomness: the hidden role of chance in life and in the markets,* 1st ed. London: Allen Lane, Penguin; 2007: 1-368.

20. Swamy S, Kupelian AS, Khasriya R, *et al.* Cross-over data supporting long-term antibiotic treatment in patients with painful lower urinary tract symptoms, pyuria and negative urinalysis. *Int Urogynecol J* 2019; 30(3): 409-14.

21. Popper KR, Hansen TE. *The two fundamental problems of the theory of knowledge.* London: Routledge; 2012.

22. Popper KR. *Objective knowledge: an evolutionary approach.* Revised ed. (reprinted with corrections and a new appendix 2). Oxford: Clarendon Press; 1979.

23. Popper K. Epistemology without a knowing subject. In: Popper K. *Objective knowledge: an evolutionary approach.* Oxford: Oxford University Press; 1973: 106-52.

24. Sestini P. Epistemology and ethics of evidence-based medicine: putting goal-setting in the right place. *J Eval Clin Pract* 2010; 16(2): 301-5.

25. Bliss M. *William Osler: a life in medicine.* Oxford: Oxford University Press; 2007.

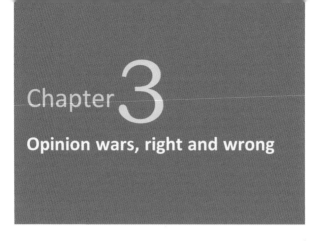

Chapter 3

Opinion wars, right and wrong

On 8th July 2020, The NHS Independent Medicines and Medical Devices Safety Review Report by Baroness Cumberlege and her team, "First do no harm" was published in the UK. We had great interest in this because we were treating patients who gave evidence to that enquiry. Chronic UTI (cUTI) is a component of the problems that follow the use of vaginal mesh. The report tells a deplorable tale of iatrogenic suffering visited on women:

> "Their experiences were harrowing. They told us of lives that had been damaged, families under immense strain, relationships destroyed, careers broken, and as a result financial ruin, with no income, many lost their homes, and faced their children being taken into care."

The enquiry describes a corrupted health care system that is deaf to inconvenient facts, particularly when those are reported by patients:

> "We heard about the failure of the system to acknowledge when things go wrong for fear of blame and litigation. There is an institutional and professional resistance to changing practice even in the face of mounting safety concerns. There can be a culture of dismissive and arrogant attitudes that only serve to intimidate and confuse. For women there is an added dimension — the widespread and wholly unacceptable labelling of so many symptoms as 'normal' and attributable to 'women's problems'."

This pleads for much soul-searching by our professions over our receptiveness to problems with our practice, particularly when patients bear witness.

But that is not all, there persists a difficulty with resistance to the critical influence of science particularly when it challenges accepted practice. We have a history of rejecting new knowledge for too long after exemplary evidence beseeched change. Gabriel Miller has provided some excellent examples on Medscape (https://www.medscape.com/features/slideshow/medical-break throughs#page=1):

- Antiseptic handwashing.
- Incubators for neonates.
- Balloon angioplasty.
- Virus aetiology of cancer.
- *Helicobacter pylori.*
- Prion disease.
- Pathogenic bacteria.
- Mendel's heredity.
- Cancer immunotherapy.
- Sport-related brain injury.

Patients suffered needlessly. Today, the causative attitudes are better understood and explained by human cognitive conditioning and group culture, but that does not excuse it.

The management of cUTI has not escaped this phenomenon, where new findings, with implications for patients with life-changing symptoms, have been resisted by a profession that is avowedly scientific, patient-focused and boasts evidence-based practice. The consequences for the patients may be damaging, but getting that recognised is a Herculean task. Because, in this book we present so much that may be new, we felt that there were good reasons to scrutinise this matter, as we experienced it, when trying to alert our profession to problems with cystitis protocols. It may help to understand the sophistry that could be used to defend the status quo. Perhaps an exposé of flawed arguments may clear the path to legitimise a call to re-examine the accepted approaches to cystitis.

Our regulatory bureaucracies separate authority from the responsibility of looking after the patients. It is a system built without feedback loops. The guideline producers are not accountable for the consequences of their decisions. However, practising clinicians must answer simultaneously, to the patients and to masters auditing compliance with these guidelines. This situation can force clinicians, caring for patients who have failed to respond to best practice recommendations, into alarming, ethical dilemmas, salted by legitimate fears of professional censure. The authors of the practice directives are not going to be confronted by such patients, so conflict is inevitable and dodgy disputation is bound to surface.

Michael Shermer's book, *The Believing Brain* [1], provides an excellent analysis of the cognitive processes that oppose change, which he encapsulated when he set out the theme of the book:

> "We form our beliefs for a variety of subjective, personal, emotional, and psychological reasons in the context of environments created by family, friends, colleagues, culture, and society at large; after forming our beliefs we then defend, justify, and rationalize them with a host of intellectual reasons, cogent arguments, and rational explanations. Beliefs come first, explanations for beliefs follow." [1]

Much quasi academic argument has nothing to do with the science; it is instead the defence of belief come hell or high water. This may manifest as pseudoscepticism, a serious menace [2] that has brought such bother to victims of UTI. Marco Truzzi provided us with an excellent analysis when he described pseudosceptics as demonstrating the following [3]:

- Denying when only doubt has been established.
- Double standards in the application of criticism; exaggerating faults in an opponent's evidence whilst understating their own.
- The tendency to discredit rather than investigate.
- Presenting insufficient evidence or proof.
- Assuming criticism requires no burden of proof.
- Making unsubstantiated counter-claims.
- Making counter-claims based on plausibility rather than empirical evidence.
- Suggesting that doubtful evidence provides grounds for completely dismissing a claim.

To him, true scepticism, had the following characteristics:

- Acceptance of doubt when neither assertion nor denial has been established.
- No burden of proof to take an agnostic position.
- Agreement that the corpus of established knowledge must be based on what is proved, but recognising its incompleteness.
- Even-handedness in requirement for proofs, whatever their implication.
- Accepting that a failure of a proof in itself proves nothing.
- Continuing examination of the results of experiments even when flaws are found.

(From https://rationalwiki.org/wiki/Pseudoskepticism.)

A sketch might depict an armchair critic, uninvolved in the graft; opining *ad hoc*, evidence-free interpretations; overstating academic minutiae; puffing his erudition; and disparaging the researcher. An image close to the truth. Empirical science was designed to overcome cognitive bias; we received an education in this. Why should we be forgiven for neglecting those skills whilst our patients come to harm?

There is much modern writing about belief and disbelief [1, 4]. Two attitudes dominate the literature; denialism and cognitive dissonance. The first features in the conflicts over evolution, the Holocaust, vaccination, AIDS aetiology and climate change. **Denialism** is the obstinate rejection of well-established empirical facts to avoid psychologically uncomfortable truths. We should not have expected to address denialism here, but we witnessed the techniques deployed to reject worrying data signalling serious problems with urinalysis accuracy.

Here is a selection of the denialist techniques used to obstruct these warnings:

- If some study data failed to endorse our proposition, the entirety was rejected, ignoring all other evidence: doubt about one thing, justified refutation of everything; thus minor matters of uncertainty were over-interpreted and granted excessive influence.

- Some insisted that we provide incontrovertible proof; but that is a prerogative of mathematics and logic. It has no place in the biological sciences, which collect evidence, building models that approximate the truth with the probability of accuracy increasing as data accumulate. We found that colleagues would dismiss what was probable because it was "unproven"; demanding impossible standards of evidence.

- Non-RCT data were disallowed. A RCT is the final step in a protracted chain of discovery. It is an expensive undertaking. The grant bodies rightly demand substantial, empirical evidence before agreeing to fund a trial. Those data are not less valid for being upstream of a RCT, otherwise the funders would not ask for them.

- There was much use of rhetoric that implied problems with our research without ever spelling it out. Thus, the words "controversial", "maverick", "eccentric", "questionable", "contentious", "disputed", "dubious" ricocheted around us. These seemed to absolve our opponents from reading the peer-reviewed published papers.

- Our patients often describe experiencing the flat denial "It is my opinion and that is the end of it". The Cumberlege report relates similar stories.

- When we first warned of a potentially harmful urinalysis problem, a senior colleague rejected the data because they were reported in conference abstracts; later it was because they were PhD theses, and ultimately our peer-reviewed publications were refused because we were the authors. Thus, the bar kept rising, the posts moving and the rules changing. A more common example is the rejection of data because they were not collected according to procedures approved by a regulatory bureaucratic process. Why do we entrust such systems to so much arbitrary, unchecked influence? The arguments were used to deny the urinalysis problem whilst justifying refusal to explore the evidence; an archetypical denialist strategy; shoot the messenger.

Why should we condone this? We are clinicians with scientific training; what has happened to our professions? Keith Kahn-Harris has written an interesting book *Denial: the Unspeakable Truth* [5]. His description of a rock-like intransigence makes it all the more depressing that denialism should have infected medicine.

Cognitive dissonance [6, 7] is a more common occurrence that is a powerful influence on the reasoning of knowledgeable, committed and caring clinicians. Matthew Syed relates a tragic medical occurrence in *Black Box Thinking* [4] and Jonathan Haidt in *The Righteous Mind* [8] covers the psychology well. Cognitive dissonance describes the experience of confronting evidence that contradicts our beliefs. It generates some mental anguish which causes us to take steps to alleviate our distress by seeking to refute what troubles us. If the unwelcome evidence is solid, we resort to sophistry and logical fallacies to defend our circumstance. As Haidt points out, our reactions are likely to be immediate, founded in our emotional consciousness and less influenced by cooler intellectual leavening. It is the rapid nature of the riposte that is a hallmark; something that must be familiar to many thinking clinicians.

Observing the discussions at a medical conference is educative for reasons differing from the organisers' intentions. A scientific forum is not a court of law; we are not there to impress our colleagues with our Cicero-like rhetorical skills; we are supposed to be seeking truth. Sadly, quick-fire, specious repartee is applauded; not so, thoughtful, data-informed, considered responses that enlighten. There are some accepted truths; shibboleths which only the foolhardy would question. Attend an industry sponsored session and you will be regaled by a "key opinion leader" whose paid retention is conditional on a positive sales result [9]. Look closely at the conference and note how the society elders are absent from the scientific sessions; they are attending committee meetings. Thus, the young and aspiring are left to present without experienced, senior contributions to the discussions.

It pays to understand the ordinance of this culture and the primary weapon is the logical fallacy. Jonathan Haidt made the point well that our approach to ideas are invariably, emotionally instinctive of the friend or foe kind; we are fiendishly loyal to our beliefs. To be influenced by sober reason we have to interact with others. Critical scrutiny and inquisition are the essence of science. Events where questions are prevented or reduced are time wasting. A keynote address without questions sets a bad example.

Asking a question is not a simple matter. Even senior clinicians can be apprehensive and discouraged by timidity. Lacking confidence and doubting ourselves, we fear revealing our deficiencies; should we make fools of ourselves? A good chairman protects time for questions, leading in with a single question. A brilliant chairman asks the "stupid" question everyone is thinking. A deficient chairman announces that there is no time for questions; that is not science; for science to thrive discussion must abound.

In 2014 our commissioners sought to close our clinical service, presumably because we worked outside guidelines. We offered to present ourselves for ruthless interrogation about our science and the evidential foundations of our practice. A date was set but the meeting was cancelled, without explanation. Nevertheless, in 2015 we were decommissioned, albeit temporarily. In 2016 a review of our service by the Royal College of Physicians did not address the science and its implications, despite these motivating all of our practice methods. The Yale and Harvard behavioural scientist Chris Argyris long ago identified the pervasiveness of undiscussables in our organisations [10, 11]. These are matters that we all recognise but avoid discussing because of discomfiture. They may be symptoms of the failure to listen that the 2020 Cumberlege review addressed.

Logical fallacies involve distorted reasoning. They are specious but plausible arguments, which closer scrutiny exposes to be deceptive imposters. They are many and ubiquitous; study of any of the websites addressing the subject (https://sites.google.com/site/skepticalmedicine/logical-fallacies) will enrich our professional and personal lives. Here we are going to discuss the important fallacies that we encountered.

Before we go further, it may help to restate the situation that caused these problems: our concern, drawn from empirical evidence, was that the tests for UTI, urinary dipstick and urine culture, were defective, incapable of excluding

UTI and that culture and genomic studies were not identifying the causative pathogen. We argued that the best indicators of UTI were symptoms and signs, and that the only current validated surrogate test for UTI was microscopy of immediately fresh, unspun, and unstained urine using a haemocytometer to count the white blood cells.

We treated our patients on this science and evolved a protocol that used protracted courses of first-generation, narrow-spectrum, urinary antibiotics combined with the urinary disinfectant methenamine. We published a description of this method [12] and a proof of concept cross-over study [13] but insisted that wider adoption must wait on the RCT that we were proposing. Our question to our colleagues was always "These tests are proven wrong so what are you going to do about it?" Too often, the reply was a tsunami of logical fallacies and our ensuing adventures came to be called the "dipstick wars".

The logical fallacies

This is not an exhaustive list but describes the fallacies that we met in our circumstances. An enormous amount of time is wasted with logical fallacies and we can all lapse into their use if we are not vigilant. The antidote is to speak to the data or from the data.

The Grand Silence

The Grand Silence — we borrow this term from Benedictine monasticism, where it has excellent intentions and is a golden idea. However, in this context it is a manifestation of Chris Argyris' organisational undiscussables [11]. A conspicuous serious problem is carefully ignored by all concerned. If we say nothing, we avoid engagement and dodge responsibility. You may have a question: "Here's the problem, there is the evidence, we do this, what would you do instead?" You cannot extract a response, certainly nothing in writing; instead you are fed the cliché, "we should meet". The meeting happens after much delay, drifts off subject, overruns and defers pending collection of data [14]. That sullen silence can outlast your retirement.

Appeal to the stone

Appeal to the stone — a critic dismisses your argument as nonsense, without offering evidence for this. Prevailing beliefs are reaffirmed with absolute certitude, refusing all doubt. The stubborn rejection of intellectual engagement is effective as it is intimidating. Blocking statements like "I just do not agree with you" or "Well I just believe" are examples, as is the stonewalling by enthusiasts when asked for evidence; all infuriating. Opinions are worthless without the justification of supporting evidence. Are we entitled to evidence-free beliefs about patient care? It must be admitted that some patients, their families and friends may also hold specious unshakable convictions about tests and treatments.

Ad hominem

Ad hominem — when critics are unable to support their position with reason and evidence they resort to the personal abuse of their opponent. The corridors fill with insults, gossip, rumours, innuendo and lies. Do not think that our leaders are any less enthusiasts for this sport. Being the target is uncongenial, but time and experience will neuter this fluff; the last redoubt of the intellectually bankrupt. Do not be provoked, stick to the science and couch your responses as questions of the form "What would you do instead and why?" Do not mock your opponent; it is not justified and it diminishes you. Do not respond by using *ad hominem* arguments yourself. Your critic may be a duck-wit but it has nothing to do with the science.

Hasty generalisation

Daniel Kahneman's [15] book *Thinking, Fast and Slow* is an important read. It describes the work by him and the late Amos Tversky that contributed to Daniel Kahneman, a psychologist, being awarded the 2002 Nobel Memorial Prize in Economic Sciences for the prospect theory, which displaced economics' equivalent of the MSU culture, the expected utility theory. Amos Tversky, also a psychologist, had died prematurely in 1996 from melanoma. Their story, described by Michael Lewis in *The Undoing Project* [16], is a moving, fascinating read.

Daniel Kahneman describes human cognition as having two systems of thought: "fast thinking" (system 1), which is impulsive, automatic, intuitive; and "slow thinking" (system 2) which is effortful, reflective and studious. The fast thinking system has evolutionary advantages affecting survival: run first, ask later. There are problems in that it is easy, undemanding and over-confident. System 1 can be tempered by system 2 through learning and thoughtful assimilation of knowledge. This will provide a frame of understanding that the fast thinking may react from. It is the purpose of military training and studiousness alike. Unfortunately, building this wisdom requires work that is demanding and fatiguing. If the learning has not been achieved, the fast thinking system must feed off imagined, evanescent ideas. Because it is bombastically assured, it is capable of massive blunders. Some people live their lives through fast thinking whereas others are reserved and diffident disciples of system 2; there is a spectrum in between.

By definition system 1 generates on-the-spot abstractions brimming with rectitude. If the person using system 1 is ill-informed, their overbearing pronouncements may verge on the barmy, but they will lack insight, and free of doubt, defend their proposition tenaciously. Thus, we have the logical fallacy of the **hasty generalisation** and it is a most delinquent aberration, a bungling incompetent. We all do this; "Turn left"; "It's all the government's fault"; "It's all in her mind". The Benedictine Grand Silence might be a suitable and welcome antidote. Another remedy might be a habit of always binding our opinions with references to the evidence.

Beware then, the loquacious opinion fabricator. These most intelligent overbearing characters disdain the toil of practical science, nor do they burn the library candle. Posing as theoreticians, they munificently expound their intellectual contrivances. Please, do not feed them alcohol. Their system 2 stores are barren, smart rhetoric is not enough; no graft, no substance.

Appeal to ignorance

Appeal to ignorance — the absence of evidence is not the same as evidence of absence. "There are no data from a RCT, so your proposition is wrong", is a fallacy. Ignorance about a proposition says nothing about its truth. Explanatory arguments "You haven't proved that it isn't menopausal" claim an unsubstantiated opinion until proved false. Data predating a RCT are not less valid prior to the RCT. The studies that discredited tests for UTI were not from RCTs but they proved the case. It is correct to build a case from all available evidence expressing your beliefs as probable inferences that have evolved as knowledge accumulates.

In this book we provide much evidence in support of the proposition that there is significant error in the guidelines. There is a substantial body of correlative evidence which crowds the first rung of Pearl's ladder [17] (*v. infra*). We have also populated the second rung with interventions in abundance. We have two studies that serve the counterfactual rung, one more rigorous than the other [12, 13]. Because we have not finished on the third rung, i.e. accomplished the RCT, many will claim that there is no need to review guideline policies. This is the fallacy coined by John Locke (1632-1704), "*argumentum ad ignorantiam*", aka argument from ignorance.

Many still attribute placebo group changes to psychosomatic effects. As an example; because we did not have placebo data, some of our seniors assumed that psychosomatic disease had not been excluded and our patients should be managed accordingly.

A placebo acts to protect the blind. Changes in the placebo group reflect the natural history of the disease and regression to the mean. The Hawthorne experiments, that sired psychosomatic explanations, were discredited as fabrications long ago [18] and nowadays the science tells us that a psychosomatic placebo response is trivial [19, 20].

As an aside, we have fought the conjecture that cUTI is a psychosomatic disease for so long. Once a clinical psychologist complained that our patients were married to a biological explanation of their disease, unsurprising when biology is the crux.

Appeal to tradition, a bandwagon, common practice or popular opinion

Appeal to tradition, a bandwagon, common practice or popular opinion — a colleague, presented with evidence that the methods used to exclude UTI are wrong, concludes that there is no need to change because everyone else practises similarly. Bandwagons can influence practice and clinical governance may be co-opted to defend this. Those in power may lack skills needed to assimilate conflicting evidence, so they defer to common practice. "Everyone knows", or "literally nobody disagrees" are classic persuader phrases used in this context. Whether right or wrong this is a false justification. We are required to rely on the science; medicine is supposed to be a scientific discipline.

Appeal to authority

Appeal to authority — this is seen in the use of the expert witness, the key opinion leader and bumptious seniority. Agreeing with an expert does have a reassuring attraction. Look at the influence of our surfeit of expert panel recommendations. When it comes to UTI, science shows the guidelines to be wrong. Regardless, we are coerced into obeying them. We may be refused the option to question or criticise because of our limitations, being insufficiently knowledgeable to doubt legitimately.

Being conversant with practice rules and protocols shields us from the need to understand the subject, as with rote learning. The scientific discipline of probing questions and expository answers will demonstrate this. Rules will never be sufficient; they are bound to be contradictory because human biology is diverse and randomly combinatory. The idea that we should all be practising similarly according to a decreed ordinance is delusional as it is unscientific. It is a fact that with cystitis the slogan, "We practice evidence-based medicine; we follow NICE guidelines" is an oxymoron.

Linked to appeals to authority is **appeal to belief**; "in my opinion" even if spoken authoritatively is no scientific statement. Implying esoteric, privileged knowledge conferred through professional stature "in my professional opinion" is no less inappropriate. **Opinion stated as fact** is of a similar breed and a lazy habit. The Columbia University theoretical physicist, Brian Greene, makes the point: "There are questions that have right and wrong answers as opposed to opinions, and we've unfortunately come to a place where many people don't make that distinction" (https://www.xpert.chat/p/brian-greene).

We are desensitised by exposure to the strident opinion pieces that fill our media. History shows that our opinions are usually wrong; we must always ask, "What is the evidence?" If you hear someone start with "In all my years of experience", run for the lifeboats, the ship is holed.

There are also the darker arts of forcing beliefs and opinions by threatening income; employment stability; cold-shouldering; group exclusion and professional licence loss. These penalties make no difference to the facts of the scientific data; that is the beauty of empirical science.

An organisation calls in external consultants to advise on a problem. The consultants present credentials that provide a patina of knowledgeable authority [21]. Their advice is provided, but evidence for their opinions is undiscussed as there is none. The organisation pursues the guidance to the letter, impatiently rebuffing all dissent, including warnings from those doing the job. Eventually, the recommended changes have to be revoked. There are important philosophical and scientific explanations for the high likelihood of these reversals and they go right back to Aristotle [18, 22-25]. What is the probability that a person not doing the job and not in the organisation knows what to do? We never know if we know best; it is a myth that we can describe best practice. Instead, that most precious attribute, practical wisdom, should be recognised and revered [26].

Appeal to consequences

Appeal to consequences — probability theory makes it clear that making predictions that you do not plan to test is a fool's errand. Complex biological systems would confound Cassandra. A property of long-tailed distributions is that the tail events are random and unpredictable. Appeal to consequences frequently predict tail events: ignoring urine cultures will lead to an antimicrobial resistance (AMR) explosion; treating women with chronic symptoms is a pathway without end; treating these women properly will cause unacceptable side effects. In all these cases, the empirical data showed the opposite. Do not make predictions that you will not test, but do keep meticulous outcome data.

We admit it! Sometimes a prediction of a long-tail event proves correct but beware of the gambler's seduction by random chance success. Ask "How many other predictions in this set were found false?"

The fallacy crops up in medicine in the form: "If you are allowed to say that, doctors will start spreading mayhem". Occasionally we have attracted the Athenian criticism of corrupting the youth, aka junior doctors. The contemporary faddish "cancel culture" shows how this error can mutate into a toxic delusion. The UK Free Speech Union, during the 2020 COVID-19 pandemic (https://freespeechunion.org/letter-to-ofcom-threatening-a-judicial-review/), alerted us all to the media suppressing criticism of the science that had informed government policy. We should tell the truth and leave our compatriots to decide for themselves. We do not know what the consequences will be.

Begging the question

Begging the question — this is a misnomer arising from a mistaken translation from Aristotle's Greek. It has nothing to do with the sententious cliché, "That begs the question". This fallacy occurs when someone holds a belief and draws a conclusion from it without evidence for the belief. An example: "A UTI is defined as a culture of $\geq 10^5$ cfu/ml of a known urinary pathogen, so a negative culture means no UTI". A patient provided us with an excellent illustration using a Socratic syllogism:

Premise 1: Negative tests = no infection.
Premise 2: The patient's tests are negative.
Conclusion: The patient has no infection.

But Socrates said the first premise MUST be fact for the syllogism to hold. Wishing it were true does not make it so.

Question begging abounds in medicine because of the ubiquity of definitions. The classic is to define a disease in terms of a test, not the pathophysiology: "The urodynamic study was normal so the patient has a normal stable bladder". At a glance it appears reasonable, but it is nonsense.

Evidence validating the urodynamic study is omitted. In fact, a committee defined the stable bladder referencing the urodynamic study alone; but by what authority? Diagnosing IC on cystoscopic findings of glomerulations is similarly question begging and fallacious.

Special pleading

Special pleading — an excuse is offered as a counter-argument to the proposition: "The culture is the best we have"; "We are only following guidelines"; "We don't have time or resources"; "We don't have a microscope"; "AMR might happen"; "I don't understand". None of these change the facts and are no substitute for coherent, data driven reasoning.

One of our band was having a postgraduate degree viva. A clinical microbiologist examiner objected to a chapter summarising the previous science, insisting it be changed by arguing that it challenged the whole clinical microbiological provision for UTI. The candidate was instructed to limit the scope of the findings to the patients of our service alone, despite the fact that the substance of the chapter reported data from other centres on different populations. This is an example of special pleading, appeal to common practice, appeal to the stone, appeal to consequences and appeal to authority (it was an examination viva). The fallacies often come in bike gangs.

The story shows how cognitive dissonance motivates censorship of data when they ought to be reported and when doubts about practice should be aired.

Special pleading will also crop up when we seek to shift the blame. "You should have done x, y or z" is surprisingly intimidating and can generate considerable anxiety. Do not be conned; ask what is the evidence for this? By what authority do they make this claim?

Straw man argument

Straw man argument — this technique puts up a different proposition and attacks that instead. We described the deficiencies in urine culture; a

59

colleague criticised us on his conjecture that we would not treat urosepsis. These were different matters, tenuously linked and the straw man was a false assumption. Appealing to the risk of AMR to justify not treating an infected patient is a straw man argument that belittles the crux of the matter, which is the infection.

Be aware that the fallacy occurs when regulatory bureaucracies act against dissidents by searching for unrelated misdeeds to punish. This was brilliantly dissected, for our times, by Arthur Miller in *The Crucible* [27]. Thus, we have NHS martinets hounding luckless staff [28] because they do not agree.

Fallacies of prejudice

Fallacies of prejudice — if we like or agree with a person, we tend to accept their arguments readily, not so given the converse. If you are a dissenter, you will antagonise people making them less open to your case. Emotion influences our intuitions; thus, race, gender, disablement, age and more will affect our receptiveness to what patients or colleagues say. Beware of the natural, instinctive antagonism to the patient who has not improved or worse, deteriorated. Patients with cUTI respond slowly with many upsets along the way; all parties must forebear.

Moving the goal posts

Moving the goal posts — related to this is the "**no true Scotsman**" fallacy. It is common, exhausting and frustrating. You answer a criticism by presenting legitimate data. The critics respond by stipulating revised criteria that must apply for them to be persuaded. The no true Scotsman fallacy uses incremental demands for greater purity of evidence. We did many experiments and data analyses prompted solely because our scrutineers kept demanding new stipulations; it is so frustrating as are so many of these fallacies.

There is an interesting sequel to our experience of this. We saw no alternative but to conduct the experiments necessary to answer these changing demands. So, today we have a library of data that refute most *ad hoc* counter-arguments. We must own up to appreciating the helpfulness of this.

The estimable Cleghorn Professor of Management Studies at McGill University, Henry Mintzberg, describes how committees tend to defer awkward matters, repetitively, between meetings, pending yet more data [14]. Such indecision may help explain some "Why wasn't anything done?" scandals. The habit risks losing the problem from the agenda. Our worries were so deferred and in the end our host organisation was ambushed by a patient-driven storm (https://www.leighday.co.uk/News/2015/November-2015/London-Trust-reverses-decision-to-shut-LUTS-clinic).

Cognitive biases

We must also be sensitive to cognitive biases which arise from heuristics (rules of thumb) that our brains have evolved to simplify and make sense of the complexities of the world around us. Patients who do not fit with expectations are vulnerable to the consequences. This is no small matter when about 30% lie on a long tail of exceptions to the rules. This is made worse by a fad that aspires to solve our health problems by enforcing simple rules [29]. **Confirmation bias** favours information that confirms existing belief so that studies are cherry-picked to defend urine culture omitting contrary data. The **availability heuristic** esteem ideas that readily come to mind. Because heavy infection renders tests impressively positive it creates a vivid impression and recalling this reassures us about test performance. The ready availability of psychosomatic explanations is a balm to bafflement. **Anchoring bias** is the tendency to fixate on the first things that we learn. At medical school, we were taught about the pre-eminence of urine culture and antibiotic sensitivity testing. It is extraordinarily difficult to shake our ensuing beliefs. **Attentional bias** focuses on some things whilst ignoring others; thus, AMR, coloured by catastrophising, stands out over more prosaic discussion of test deficiencies and treatment feedback loops. The **Dunning-Kruger effect** is where we consider ourselves better informed than we are and fail to recognise our limitations. We make inferences unaware of the probability laws that should temper our conjectures. Doctors pass professional stages where they choose unequivocally not to pursue research careers. Nevertheless, some continue to presume knowledge necessary to expound on research practice. Perhaps this explains the habit of interpreting RCT data without considering the prior evidence and attendant probability. Lacking insight, we are shocked when confronted with our limitations. If we do not know whether we know, "I do not know" is a safe option.

The power of consistency

It is a property of our cognition that writing down an idea will encourage belief in it [30]. Write an opinion, publish a scientific paper, guideline or directive and we will be harder to dissuade than having just thought or spoken about this. Try to challenge the veracity of a guideline with someone involved in writing it compared with those not involved. We must be alert to this tendency in ourselves.

The unknown unknowns

In February 2002, the United States Secretary of Defence, Donald Rumsfeld, responded to a journalist's question about the lack of evidence for the Iraq government supplying WMD to terrorist groups:

> "Reports that say that something hasn't happened are always interesting to me, because as we know, there are known knowns; there are things we know we know. We also know there are known unknowns; that is to say we know there are some things we do not know. But there are also unknown unknowns — the ones we don't know we don't know. And if one looks throughout the history of our country and other free countries, it is the latter category that tend to be the difficult ones."

Politics would have coloured perceptions, and this was ridiculed in the press for some time. Later, it was reappraised as an insightful, true statement, if a little convoluted. The unknown unknowns are problematic, plaguing us with random events that we cannot predict. cUTI being inchoate, must conceal numerous such snares. We have to be wary of *ad hoc* speculative explanations and accept that numerous unknowns preclude imposing guidelines. When our clinic was closed in 2015, one of the justifications put to the indignant patients was "We have to follow national guidelines". It was fictional special pleading; there were no guidelines for cUTI. It would take a crazy person to write guidelines for unknown unknowns, but we can assure you that this was proposed to us.

Tread carefully; there are probably numerous unknowns yet to be unearthed. If we go slowly we shall get there quickly.

Emotions and fallacies

Now for an undiscussable! We run a clinical email service for patients, and it is our most instructive exercise in difficult medicine. It was created originally as a telephone service to siphon in negative feedback so as to increase the selection pressure of our evolutionary method. It is stressful to administer the numerous enquiries. Difficult problems are worrying, the more so without the face-to-face contact, and some messages are disturbing. We have tested various systems but have discovered that skill and experience are needed to manage the traffic. Nowadays our most senior clinician is delegated this role.

The work generates fatigue, anxiety, frustration and exasperation aggravated by the pressure of demand and expectation. The service is primarily for side effects, treatment failures and complications so dissatisfaction flavours everything.

We rarely admit it, but despite the patients' manifest innocence, the clinician can find the content annoying, the descriptions of distress irksome and the questions unwelcome, particularly if the patients suggest treatments. It feels shameful to admit to such deficiencies in our humanity; that we can find people in need annoying. It is a reaction so contrary to what we aspire to and wish others to perceive. How can this be? These experiences have explained to us much about the anatomy of negative reactions to patients with chronic disease. Cognitive dissonance will encourage us to conceal these shameful emotions and resort to self-justifying behaviours, one of which is to blame the patient. In fact, it is just a natural aspect of the messy interactions of normal life and recognising this is half the battle.

The fundamental attribution error [31] means that we attribute unflattering personal characteristics as the cause of mistakes by others, but for ourselves we attribute external influences outside of our control; that is how we blame the patient. We project onto others attitudes and motivations that are fictional inventions of our imaginings. The sophists of psychoanalysis set a precedent by extemporising specious explanations for behaviour, thus we have "It's in the patient's mind". This category error replaces empirical evidence with inference from ideas, just as much as social science research uses interpretive methods; a practice so commonplace we fail to spot the problem.

We should not deny that it is frustrating if a treatment fails or side effects occur. The patients sense the tensions because they apologise for themselves. There is no blame to apportion, but defensiveness lurks here anyway. It would seem that worry, fear of failure, and not knowing what to do influence our reactions.

It helps us to sleep on the matter. Strive to identify a valid, pathophysiological explanation for the problem; chastened, we have fashioned our software to compel us to do so. Failing that, discuss it with a colleague; we use instant messaging for that purpose, and the group support is so helpful.

Defending the indefensible

It is a worthwhile pastime to watch the strategies by which pseudoscience and hermetics deflect critical questioning. There appear to be six levels of vindication:

- Ignore.
- Deny.
- Deploy logical fallacies.
- *Ad hominem* attack.
- Claim victimhood.
- Histrionics.

It's a potent, heady brew; see 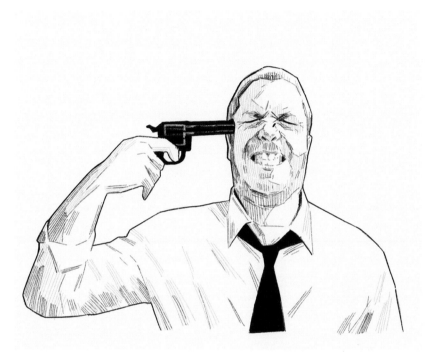 Figure 3.1 for a response.

Figure 3.1. Goalpost moving counter-strategy. *Illustration courtesy of Alex Wilby.*

We positioned our top postgraduate student under the goalposts for the next protocol acquiescence review committee (whatever) session — an enviably masterful performance. Note the subtle touch of the necktie; designed to provoke a straw man decoy argument from the compliance officers.

Postmodernism

Do not think that medicine has escaped postmodernism [32, 33]: a philosophical movement that avowedly rejects reality and reason in favour of feelings. Relativism has been around forever; "There is nothing either good or bad, but thinking makes it so" (Hamlet Act 2 Scene 2) but postmodernism has taken it to another sphere.

It has penetrated many parts of our culture and touches all of us [34]. Take the validated finding that "urinary dipsticks and culture data are misleading": mustered in opposition, we witnessed all of the following: denial by claiming victimhood because the idea offended, challenged, intimidated or alienated.

When our case survived critical scrutiny, protests were lodged claiming unfair academic and educational advantage. Evidence was rejected because the researchers were from outside professional group boundaries. Patients' opinions were disallowed for causing stress to clinicians. Appeals for change were rebuffed because they emanated from university power structures that should be opposed.

The lifeblood of learning is to question and to answer. Socrates taught this. Expository questions are indispensable to humankind, no less the answers. Postmodernist culture sanctions the appeal to the victimhood of bruised vanity as an appropriate response to a sceptical question; a wink away from the accusation of bullying, and when that arrives with its acolytes, dialogue freezes and progress dies. Look, the patients are in trouble so we must toughen up. When we cannot answer a question, we learn we do not die. For ourselves, the greatest interest is what we do not know, not what we know.

We experienced the defence of our science being reframed as having problems with another's point of view; a deviation necessitating remediation as a condition of licence revalidation. The latter horror, "You must be educated to our point of view or there will be consequences", seems to be an intrusion of cancel culture, or has this always been lurking in our world?

You may ask:

Q   "Did you seek remedial training?"
A   "We did indeed".
Q   "Did you learn anything?"
A   "We did learn" — use science and the Socratic method, May *et al* [35].

Q   "Did this make a difference to your revalidation chances?"
A   "No, it did not because we still held with the scientific findings".

This is like Kafka. Given the fear and fatigue it is tricky to manage; so find a mentor. For a start you could not do better than read the reference May *et al, Plato's Socratic Dialogues and the Epistemology of Modern Medicine* [35]. In using the Socratic method, we first explicate our critic's opinion and then follow with a question that presents an exception to that opinion; we next ask our opponent's view on an alternative proposition which might be a better fit. We should steer clear of didacticism, preferably feigning ignorance.

Critical empirical science exists to filter out our aberrant beliefs, but where do these come from? We may assume our rationality, but we are oblivious to the covert encroachment of cultural fads and fashions into our ideas. Thus, postmodernism instils the unconscionable into professional attitudes. Vigilance is the only protection. We should not be passive. We are exhorted to be courageous and show confidence in the power of reason and science; the Enlightenment's gift for all humanity.

References

1.   Shermer M. *The believing brain: from ghosts and gods to politics and conspiracies — how we construct beliefs and reinforce them as truths*, 1st ed. New York: Times Books; 2011: xii, 385.

2.   Shermer M. Forging doubt. *Sci Am* 2015; 312: 74.

3.   Truzzi M. On pseudo-skepticism. *Zetetic Scholar* 1987; 12/13: 2.

4.   Syed M. *Black box thinking: why most people never learn from their mistakes — but some do.* New York: Portfolio/Penguin; 2015: xi, 322.

5.   Kahn-Harris K. *Denial: the unspeakable truth.* Kendal, Cumbria: Notting Hill Editions; 2018: xi, 187.

6.   Festinger L. *Conflict, decision, and dissonance.* Stanford, California: Stanford University Press; 1964: vii, 163.

7.   Tavris C, Aronson E. *Mistakes were made (but not by me): why we justify foolish beliefs, bad decisions and hurtful acts.* London: Pinter & Martin; 2008.

8. Haidt J. *The righteous mind: why good people are divided by politics and religion*, 1st ed. New York: Pantheon Books; 2012: xvii, 419.

9. Moynihan R. Key opinion leaders: independent experts or drug representatives in disguise? *BMJ* 2008; 336(7658): 1402-3.

10. Noonan WR. *Discussing the undiscussable: a guide to overcoming defensive routines in the workplace*, 1st ed. San Francisco, California: Jossey-Bass; Chichester: John Wiley; 2007.

11. Argyris C. Making the undiscussable and its undiscussability discussable. *Public Adm Rev* 1980; 40(3): 205-13.

12. Swamy S, Barcella W, De Iorio M, *et al*. Recalcitrant chronic bladder pain and recurrent cystitis but negative urinalysis: what should we do? *Int Urogynecol J* 2018; 29(7): 1035-43.

13. Swamy S, Kupelian AS, Khasriya R, *et al*. Cross-over data supporting long-term antibiotic treatment in patients with painful lower urinary tract symptoms, pyuria and negative urinalysis. *Int Urogynecol J* 2019; 30(3): 409-14.

14. Mintzberg H. *Simply managing: what managers do and can do better*. San Francisco: Berrett-Koehler Publishers, Inc.; 2013: viii, 202.

15. Kahneman D. *Thinking, fast and slow*. London: Penguin Books; 2012.

16. Lewis M. *The undoing project: a friendship that changed the world*. London: Penguin Books; 2017.

17. Pearl J, Mackenzie D. *The book of why: the new science of cause and effect*. London: Allen Lane; 2018.

18. Stewart M. *The management myth: debunking modern business philosophy*. New York; London: W. W. Norton; 2010.

19. Hrobjartsson A, Kaptchuk TJ, Miller FG. Placebo effect studies are susceptible to response bias and to other types of biases. *J Clin Epidemiol* 2011; 64(11): 1223-9.

20. Hrobjartsson A, Gotzsche PC. Placebo interventions for all clinical conditions. *Cochrane Database Syst Rev* 2010; 1: CD003974.

21. Stewart M. *The management myth: why the experts keep getting it wrong*, 1st ed. New York; London: W. W. Norton; 2009.

22. Mintzberg H, Ahlstrand BW, Lampel J. *Management? It's not what you think!* New York: AMACOM; 2010: x, 132.

23. Reeve CDC. *Aristotle on practical wisdom: Nicomachean ethics VI*. Cambridge, MA: Harvard University Press; 2013.

24. Hooks B. *Teaching critical thinking: practical wisdom*. London: Routledge; 2010.

25. Schwartz BS, Sharpe K. *Practical wisdom: the right way to do the right thing*. London: Penguin Putnam Inc; 2011.

26. Bondi L. *Towards professional wisdom: practical deliberation in the people professions.* Farnham: Ashgate; 2011.

27. Miller A. *The crucible.* London: Heinemann; 1967.

28. Malone-Lee J. Dharmasena case: responsibility takes precedence over accountability. *BMJ* 2015; 350: h1131.

29. Malde S, Palmisani S, Al-Kaisy A, Sahai A. Guideline of guidelines: bladder pain syndrome. *BJU Int* 2018; 122(5): 729-43.

30. Cialdini RB. *Influence: science and practice*, 5th ed. Boston: Pearson Education; 2009: xii, 259.

31. Ross L. From the fundamental attribution error to the truly fundamental attribution error and beyond: my research journey. *Perspect Psychol Sci* 2018; 13(6): 750-69.

32. Frost DP. Medicine, postmodernism, and the end of certainty. Complex systems result in a new kind of fundamental uncertainty. *BMJ* 1997; 314(7086): 1045.

33. Hodgkin P. Medicine, postmodernism, and the end of certainty. *BMJ* 1996; 313(7072): 1568-9.

34. Hicks SRC. *Explaining postmodernism: skepticism and socialism from Rousseau to Foucault.* Ockham's Razor; 2011.

35. May J, Baum M, Bewley S. Plato's Socratic dialogues and the epistemology of modern medicine. *J Roy Soc Med* 2010; 103(12): 484-9.

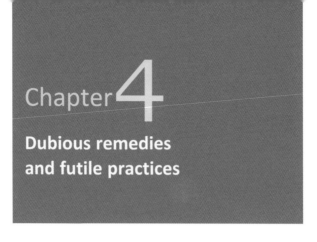

Chapter 4

Dubious remedies and futile practices

Ideology is not theory

To avoid confusion, we must clarify some terminology. A hypothesis is a proposition that has been abducted from the assimilation of data observed by induction. The hypothesis justifies a prediction that must be true if the hypothesis is correct. Empirical science tests predictions which are thus verified or falsified. A theory is an explanation of phenomena, supported by much, widespread experimentation. The cliché "He has a theory" is misapplied, as are the faddish, evidence-free theories, that capture sociological commentary; we are too ignorant to write theories; that is for people like Charles Darwin or Alfred Russel Wallace. An idea first floats autonomously in the imagination; unless mathematical, it has to be grounded by empirical science. In medicine, ideas which escape pragmatic scrutiny can and do generate ideologies that can only be defended by rhetoric. Hence the rationalising effect of the question "What is your evidence?" To describe ideas as theory provides them with a patina of respectability. Some will thus peddle ideology as truth and inveigle us to act on it. Committees are hotbeds of such, with ideas and opinions pinging off the walls. Tragically we are enslaved to a "pompousethora" of committees. Philosophy over the last 2500 years tells us that ideas are so fickle as to be wrong over 95% of the time; hence the importance for empirical science. Freudian psychoanalysis is an archetypical ideology hawked as science. It may be uncomfortable to acknowledge this, but in our context, interstitial cystitis, mast cell activation disorder, urodynamics, bladder instillations, urethral dilation, cystodistension and much else, feed off ideological fabrications.

Doubts about procedures and treatment

We are writing about UTI, focusing on chronic recalcitrant bladder pain and recurrent cystitis. We use that term because the patients have been found to show signs of UTI when a microscope is used to examine an immediately fresh, unspun, unstained specimen of urine to count the white blood cells. They have microscopic pyuria (white blood cells in the urine) and the published scientific evidence renders UTI the standout most probable explanatory cause. It should be noted that the published evidence on pyuria indicates that any pyuria is not normal and should not be explained away. If we found no evidence of infection, an easy task if you use urinary dipsticks or cultures as your tests, then these patients would attract a diagnosis of "interstitial cystitis" or "painful bladder syndrome" or "bladder pain syndrome" (IC/PBS/BPS) [1].

Interstitial cystitis

In 1987 the National Institute of Diabetes and Digestive and Kidney Diseases (NIDDK) described a set of criteria "for research purposes", which became accepted as the diagnostic criteria for IC, without a justification on evidence. These required findings of bladder pain, urgency, glomerulations, or a Hunner's ulcer, as well as the absence of 18 exclusions. In many respects the definition was a diagnosis of exclusion. These criteria were found to be too restrictive in clinical practice, excluding 60% of cases where a painful bladder was evident [2]. This raises the legitimate question as to how was the diagnosis being achieved? What was the reference standard? In 2002 the International Continence Society (ICS) published new recommendations and proposed that IC should be renamed painful bladder syndrome (PBS). The ICS diagnosis of PBS is based on suprapubic pain related to bladder filling, day- or night-time frequency, and the absence of other obvious pathology [3]. IC was retained to describe those who had cystoscopic findings. It is bewildering that later another committee renamed this "bladder pain syndrome" (BPS); what did that add to the science? There is a common thread; groups of clinicians form committees and their opinions cluster symptoms and signs into a syndrome that may become widely adopted. The absence of evidence and a scientific foundation seem not to matter. You cannot do science by committee.

There are no published data that are helpful in describing the pathophysiology of this condition. Work on IC/PBS/BPS has been piecemeal, sporadic and lacking in any clear coherent narrative. There are numerous published ideas on the aetiology, which are usually given the status of theory despite the scarcity of hypothesis-driven critical research. There is a pressing need for a systematic, critical scrutiny of this condition, eschewing all evidence-free assumptions about infection, inflammation or immunity.

All definitions of IC/PBS/BPS stipulate a crucial step — the absence of UTI. Unfortunately, the tests used to rule out UTI cannot rule out UTI and the risk of a missed infection is substantial. There is another problem; IC/PBS/BPS is a diagnosis of exclusion; what remains having excluded all other options. This is called a "Holmesian" or "Sherlock Holmes fallacy" or "process of elimination fallacy". In *The Adventure of the Blanched Soldier* the great master opined "When you have eliminated all which is impossible, then whatever remains, however improbable, must be the truth" [4]. Shock-horror — he got it wrong! Mycroft Holmes would have corrected his brother; it is false to assume that you can eliminate ALL options unless you be a deity. Thus, IC/PBS/BPS is a Holmesian fallacy.

Whilst IC/PBS/BPS may prove to be a heterogeneous group of conditions, the evidence suggests that missed chronic UTI is a major player that demands considerable elucidation. That is not the same as claiming that all cases are infection, which is a commonly used canard. We are going to discuss a number of the treatments for IC/PBS/BPS here because many of our patients were exposed to these when in the end, they were found to have cUTI.

Quackery and its endorsement

The patients with IC/PBS/BPS/cUTI suffer terribly; their lives are broken and they are desperately vulnerable. Their symptoms are dreadful; the consequences so destructive they will do anything to seek respite and are vulnerable to opportunists. In 2019 we attended the International Urogynaecology Association (IUGA) conference in Nashville. This is promoted as a scientific conference and it is undoubtedly influential. For example, the mesh procedures were first promoted there. We approached an exhibition stand promoting a cranberry extract for cystitis (about £25 GBP for 30 tablets, dose 1 tablet a day, about £300 GBP a year). They had no evidence of efficacy to show and none for the claims that they were making. To our horror, they were promoting their own urinary dipstick test kit. We took them on; this is our territory — we know the subject well, particularly microbial adhesion chemistry which is used to spin cranberry extracts and D-mannose. The reps were ignorant of the science, new cUTI knowledge and ill-understood dipstick validation. However, they were encyclopaedias of logical fallacies. They were unable to provide a coherent reason for using their products. Our challenge was that they were selling an expensive, unproved product to a vulnerable group. Their cold indifference to the patients' plight, contempt for science, shamelessness in hyping pathetic data, and their preposterous claims was awful. What is the point of the labour of science when various organisations host such companies with these attitudes? If you surf the internet you will find many sites flogging junk to IC patients all finessed with the saccharine compassion of kitsch caring.

There are doctors who betray their education to endorse specious remedies, presumably for financial gain. Patient-support organisations flog dubious and evidence-free remedies for profit. We are insufficiently assertive in deploring these practices, which extract large costs from vulnerable people whilst informed clinicians remain silent or, worse, collude. Quackery behaves like the Lernaean Hydra; decapitation leads to immediate, multiple replacements; we must up our game and respond to this Herculean challenge.

Sontag surmise

We should like to introduce you to the "Sontag surmise" after the late Susan Sontag, the cultural critic with a tendency to extrapolate theories from a single empirical fact. Herbert Marcuse observed that "She can make a theory out of a potato skin". The Sontag surmise reigns here: a conjecture one minute is a belief the next. Without hesitation outcomes are anticipated and pre-empt the science with such energetic conviction that when the inevitable falsification happens, it is too late and the quack remedy has penetrated the market.

GAG layer and IC/PBS/BPS

If you wished to find an example of a Sontag surmise you could not do better than the GAG layer blunders. Glycosaminoglycans (GAG), also known as mucopolysaccharides, are long chains of sugar molecules that are found in the extracellular matrix all over the body and we usually meet them in mucus. Roughly, there are four types: heparan sulphate (HSGAGs), chondroitin sulphate (CSGAGs), keratin sulphate and hyaluronic acid. These names will be familiar to any IC/PBS/BPS groupie. Given that these molecules are so widely distributed in the body, it should be no surprise that we find them coating the urothelial cells of the bladder (GAG layer) which was what was described in 1986 along with the Sontag surmise that "malfunction of this layer could be involved in a spectrum of urologic diseases" [5] along with the Olympian leap that the oral agent pentosan polysulfate sodium (Elmiron®) could be prescribed to replace the defect. Chemistry showed no difference in urothelial cell GAG content between controls and IC patients [6]. Electron microscopy found GAG layers similarly intact on cells from controls and IC patients in 1993 [7]. Despite this there was no stopping it and an ideological model for IC and GAG layers was proposed and gained traction [8]. It was next reported that urinary hyaluronic acid concentrations were raised in IC with the surmise that it was leaking from the damaged urothelium [9].

Microbes will form biofilms on any water/surface interface and the normal or inflamed bladder urothelium will be covered in biofilm. Biofilms consist of bacteria and mucus. Mucus is made up in part of mucopolysaccharides which are nowadays called glycosaminoglycans, termed GAG. The microbial biofilms would make a better job of GAG layer repair than these medications.

Think about this, someone offers a theory without evidence that IC/PBS/BPS might be caused by disruption of the GAG layer of the bladder surface cells. Two sensible experiments show that this is not the case. Nevertheless, a professional juggernaut decides that the patients should be treated by restoring the non-missing GAG layer. Without evidence, this has sired an industry of oral supplementation and bladder instillations all justified by a whimsical ideology. It is not good, but the resulting suffering, harm and expense caused to the patients is reprehensible.

It must be said that the natural GAG layers have a complex biological relationship with their host cells which are constantly reabsorbing and replacing this surface mucopolysaccharide. It has a short half-life of about a day or two. In this context, replacement by instillations weekly or more does not make sense [10, 11].

Pentosan polysulfate sodium (Elmiron®)

Pentosan polysulfate sodium is similar in structure to the heparan GAGs. Its introduction was motivated by an idea; the oral administration of this drug was claimed to repair the bladder GAG layer which basic science had shown not to be deficient anyway. The manufacturers themselves admit "It is not completely understood how the drug works", but they provide seductive images of their imaginings of GAG layer defects and repair despite the fact that science contradicts this. Let us offer a similitude; GAG contains keratin sulphate; why not feed the patients powdered antlers? We have lots of them in Wiltshire.

Much of the data that were published to support pentosan polysulfate sodium lacked scientific rigour, although a placebo-controlled RCT found it ineffective in 1987 [12]. The authors wrote: "We conclude that no statistically or clinically significant effect of sodium pentosan polysulfate was found compared to placebo in patients with painful bladder disease". Scrupulously fair, the authors also said: "A significant increase in the cystoscopically determined bladder capacity in the sodium pentosan polysulfate group in protocol A was found". This nod to the contemporary infatuation with p-values is important: if you collect multiple outcomes, probability favours one or more randomly demonstrating a statistically significant effect (p<.05). Search outcomes with a p-value detector and bingo! You have efficacy despite no efficacy. This is why we should insist on a single, clinically relevant outcome measure reporting the effect size first; p-value last, if at all.

This is no pastiche; clinical researchers do this commonly. "Take this drug — it may increase your cystoscopic bladder capacity; it won't do much else but we dredged up a p-value". Thus, the diabolical, statistically significant p-value feeds off its victim.

The pentosan polysulfate sodium (Elmiron®) story is a good illustration of **regression to the mean**, which is a great way of demonstrating evidence for quack remedies. So in 1987 an open uncontrolled study of pentosan polysulfate sodium concluded: "Therefore, the study indicates that a significant number of patients with interstitial cystitis can be expected to benefit from treatment with sodium pentosan polysulfate" [13]. How can this be?

Figure 4.1 illustrates the graph of white blood cell counts (pyuria) measured at each consultation during the follow-up of a patient being

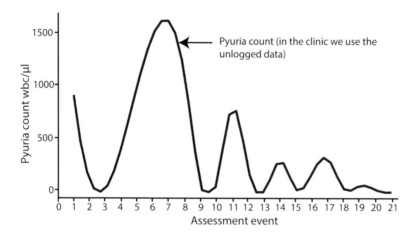

Figure 4.1. Urinary white blood cells by assessment events.

This is a damped oscillation and it is the healing pattern that we strive to achieve. However, patients recruited into trials are likely to be on a peak and the natural oscillation of the disease will provide a following trough that may not have anything to do with a therapeutic response. We must use a much more sophisticated approach to measuring outcomes than point estimates; hence, we insist on using graphs and trials without treatment. A rising count after treatment cessation is evidence against a regression effect. From a clinical management perspective, if there is a damped oscillation we know that the treatment is working and we do not change in response to the inevitable flares; this avoids cycling or shuffling of prescriptions which is good for preventing AMR.

treated for a chronic UTI. It demonstrates an archetypical pattern seen in 75% of our patients. It is called a damped oscillation and involves a series of peaks and troughs of decreasing amplitude. In this case the patient is responding so the oscillations are damping out; a patient not responding would oscillate without damping even when deteriorating (■ Figure 4.2). In recruiting patients into clinical trials we select them because they have plentiful manifestations of the disease in order to have something to measure. We are

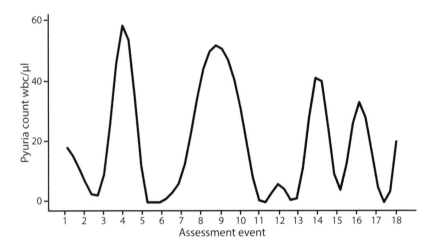

Figure 4.2. Urinary white blood cells by assessment events.

This is a worrying situation which is fortunately not so common. It is bad; the plot shows that we are not getting the condition under control and things are getting worse. The oscillations are occurring and there is no therapeutic response; on the contrary there is deterioration. However, the troughs may be used to claim benefit falsely, despite the facts of the matter. A trough may motivate the doctor to discharge the patient, reassuring that all is well. We must treat in order to see a coherent response trend overall which is a damped oscillation. An overall perspective achieved by graphing is most important. Point estimates can be so misleading.

therefore biased towards patients who are at a peak and not a trough. If we then do nothing, probability still favours the detection of a better state because the measurements will move towards the mean lying between the peaks and troughs. Thus, without proper controls, a study may detect a spurious therapeutic effect. The case in ▨ Figure 4.2 could dissemble as recovery at several points.

A RCT, done properly, will address the problem of regression to the mean. If you do not have the necessary resources, a common circumstance, you can compensate by randomly crossing patients between treatment and no treatment [14, 15]. This is a powerful and legitimate option that is built into our practice protocol. It allows us to generate evidence, from pyuria oscillations, on whether our treatments are helping or not. The quacks do not do this.

In 2015 a large RCT [16] reported as follows: "No treatment effect vs. placebo for pentosan polysulfate sodium". Then, in 2018 we learned that pentosan polysulfate sodium caused vision-threatening macular degeneration [17]. But in 2019 NICE proposed recommending pentosan because a meta-analysis of the pooled data from the clinical trials showed a statistically significant effect — $p<.05$. The uselessness of the effect size was not considered. It illustrates how barmy frequentist evidence-based medicine can be: it gives us p-value drugs exhibiting statistically significant but clinically useless effects.

This is not a happy story; Elmiron® costs about £7.90 per 100mg tablet and the dose is 100mg three times a day. It is extraordinary that it has been endorsed by regulatory and prescribing authorities. There is something wrong with our systems; we have to do better than this.

Bladder instillations

The bladder instillation quagmire owes itself to the fatuous proposition that you can replace the non-missing GAG layer by instilling GAG components into the bladder. Sodium hyaluronate, a salt of hyaluronic acid, is marketed as Cystistat® or Hyacyst®. Chondroitin sulphate is marketed as Uracyst® or

Gepan®. Then hyaluronic acid has been combined with chondroitin to give us iAluril®. Parsons' solution is a combination of lidocaine and heparin. Parsons was the person who proposed the damaged GAG layer idea [5]. Dimethyl sulfoxide (DMSO) is a detergent and drug mule that transports pharmaceuticals through cell membranes. It claims palliative analgesic properties that are mightily underwhelming [18]. Finally, we have lidocaine and simple sodium bicarbonate, marketed as Cystilieve™ which is a combination of a local anaesthetic and the well-known alkalinising agent.

Given the basic science, we must wonder at what these instillations achieve. The GAG layer on the urothelial cells of IC patients is found, by electron microscopy, to be present and correct [7]. The animal studies conducted on GAG layers shows that instilled hyaluronic acid and heparin do not replace or bind to the urothelial GAG layer. Chondroitin binds to ulcerated urothelium but not to normal surface cells [19]. What that might achieve is unknown, although the potential for a Sontag surmise as an *ad hoc* rescue should not be overlooked; "It eases your ulcerations".

The data on bladder instillations illustrates another consequence of judging efficacy on a p-value. A widespread outcome measure is the Interstitial Cystitis Symptom Index (ICSI) [20]. The paper explaining the validation of this score is short on data but it is possible to work out that normal persons tend to score between 0 and 3. There are numerous papers which report the p<.05 significant effects but they do not dwell on the micro effect size. For example [21]: a comparison of two instillations reported ICSI scores after instillations (1) Mean = 6.45, SD = 3.00 and (2) Mean = 6.67, SD = 3.06. After 6 months of treatment the patients were still sick. The authors reported a statistically significant effect, albeit useless, and there was no mention of regression to the mean.

There is a great deal of shoddy work: p-value fishing [22]; absence of controls [23]; reporting the change in symptoms score (p<.05) without admitting to the many residual symptoms at study end [24]; claiming an effect without considering regression to the mean [25]; using unvalidated outcome measures [26]; declaring an effect despite a p=.15 result [27]; "comparing" two active agents by reporting the within group changes; ignoring the insignificant between group differences and failing to acknowledge that the patients were still sick [28].

There have been some meta-analyses; one cheerfully optimistic report observed "Long-term and placebo-controlled studies were few" referencing one placebo-controlled trial [29]. Another favoured botulinum toxin injections and reported pentosan polysulfate sodium as helping frequency and urgency when the patients complained of bladder pain [30]; another reported five controlled but 14 uncontrolled trials [31]. Finally, a Cochrane review found no evidence of efficacy [32], by which time we had lost the will to live. Given the widespread use of these products, we are entitled to ask, what is the point of the rituals of systematic review?

These treatments are ludicrous; they do not work, they are expensive, painful and they raise false hopes in the patients. They should not be used and we should ask how it is that they saw the light of day in the first place.

Bacteriophages

Bacteriophages are viruses that parasitise bacteria and use them to reproduce thereby killing the microbe. They are tempting options for the non-antibiotic treatment of bacterial infection. They have been trying to get them to work for cystitis in Tbilisi, Georgia, for a long time but so far no joy. A negative trial report used 30 words of fashionably arcane prose to say "ineffective": "Intravesical bacteriophage therapy was non-inferior to standard-of-care antibiotic treatment, but was not superior to placebo bladder irrigation, in terms of efficacy or safety in treating UTIs in patients undergoing TURP" — Amen [33]. There are millions of phages, all most choosy about the bacteria that they will attack. Thus, to treat UTI we must know the causative species. Currently, phage selection rests on urine culture isolates that do not identify causation. The phage story, which periodically sees a flurry of enthusiasm, is a good example of the blind alleys that the false assumptions about causation lead us to.

The herbalists arrive

At the end of the nineteenth century there was considerable interest in using organic acids to shift the pH of the urine as a means of treating or preventing UTI. Methenamine hippurate was a product of these endeavours. It was noted that cranberries appeared to have potential because their benzoic acid content increased urinary concentrations of the bacteriostatic hippuric acid [34]. However, cranberries had no bacteriostatic effect on *Escherichia coli* [35]. The hippuric acid proposition was subsequently refuted so people set out in search of another explanation for the presumed properties of cranberries. That was when it was reported that cranberry juice inhibited the adhesion of bacteria to the urothelial cells, which is a key step in the process of infection [36]. So from that moment the story was that cranberry worked by its anti-adhesion properties; there was no stopping it. In 2016 we saw the publication of an excellent RCT that showed that cranberry juice had no effect on bacteriuria and no therapeutic effect; it was in truth useless [37]. NICE had to rescind its recommendation to use it, but why were they doing this in the first place?

However, remember the Hydra simile; cranberry has risen from the ashes! Step forward proanthocyanidins. These have been shown *in vitro* to achieve a dose-dependent partial inhibition of the adherence of microbes to urothelial cells. It is not an absolute inhibition [38]. However, bioavailability studies find that the polyphenols least well-absorbed from the intestines are the proanthocyanidins [39]. Proanthocyanidins were the subject of a recidivist study comparing three active herbal groups, without a control, and crazy statistics [40]. Marketed as Ellura® and Utiva®, these are expensive products that are promoted with extravagant claims and without valid efficacy data.

D-Mannose

E. coli has been the microbe most studied in research on UTI. It is much stated that *E. coli* parasitise urothelial cells by first adhering to the cell surface, achieved by molecules on their fimbriae, threads or tentacles, binding to receptors on the cells. Some of these receptors are made from oligomannose glycoproteins containing mannose but others contain different carbohydrate sugar moieties. The former are termed "mannose sensitive" and the latter "mannose resistant". The D isomer of mannose binds to mannose-sensitive receptors, a potential mechanism to competitively inhibit the binding of the fimbrial adhesion molecules at the tip of type one fimbriae. These facts are promoted widely whilst omitting that other binding receptors are unaffected by D-Mannose. Why spoil a good story? D-Mannose, suitably costly, is sold to prevent UTI in animals and humans, but we don't know if it does this.

Nobody has bothered to conduct pharmacokinetic studies to measure the relationship between oral dose and urinary concentration. It was only in 2018 that a urinary assay was published [41]. One RCT has been accomplished but the outcome was based on cultures of 10^3 cfu/ml that has been discredited [42]. D-Mannose compared to nitrofurantoin 50mg daily performed similarly, but these agents may alter the culture properties of the urine regardless of symptoms. The devil in UTI clinical trials is the culture-based primary outcome measures, which are proven duds.

Patient accounts report that D-Mannose helps ease symptoms in some. We note that many formulations include an alkali, a useful symptom palliative. Watch out for that trick; why pay for overpriced potassium citrate? Some patients describe benefit, others do not. The biochemistry means that at best the effect must be partial.

Biofilm busters

Part of the story following the identification of biofilms inside urothelial cells or on their surfaces in 2003 [43] illustrates another contra-scientific tendency. Here is a quotation from a website addressing cUTI:

"Natural biofilm busters: biofilm busters are super nutrients that help dissolve the sticky biofilm of bacteria within the bladder and body. Additionally some may disrupt the formation of biofilms by

83

preventing bacterial communication and growth (known as quorum sensing). There are various formulations and your alternative practitioner must decide which one(s) are best for you. Other existing health conditions must always be taken into account."

Another Sontag surmise in an extrapolative leap: biofilms on the bladder? No problem, dial up the busters. Biofilms cover all of our surfaces and are part of our normal physiology. We have complex, health-giving mutualist relationships with numerous microbes, many living in biofilms. For example, the corneas at the front of our eyes are covered by biofilm. We must assume that an effective biofilm buster would risk blindness.

If you look deeper into this, you will find many sites making wild, unsubstantiated claims for remedies which have never undergone experimental evaluation. The claimants imply privileged knowledge that licenses them to express their opinions as fact.

Other "natural" remedies

We should deal with other similar "naturals" whilst we are here. These all draw on some rootless idea adopted to concoct a material application without science. Those with relevant vested interest will state trenchantly that the remedies work and fabricate a vaguely plausible myth to explain why. Believers will join the bandwagon and patients feel obliged to try, just in case they miss an opportunity. Have you ever wondered why the herbalists offer so much choice? Keep trying but keep paying: oil of oregano, colloidal silver, zinc, uva ursi, grapefruit seed extract, dietary manipulation, marshmallow root tea and other teas, herbs, salt, garlic/allicin, aloe vera, with many more to follow; forget them, save your money — if there were evidence for efficacy we should have explored them. Acupuncture and homeopathy are similarly blighted and unable to show a useful effect in clinical trials.

At this point it may be sensible to address some other options that our patients tell us that they have been exposed to. Chinese herbs, hyperbaric oxygen, prebiotics and probiotics are all hawked to vulnerable people willing to try anything. We have little doubt that this list will continue to be increased just to sell another nostrum to be tried just in case. The merchants are capitalising on the patients' suffering. There is never evidence. Those promoting these should be challenged to provide justification and condemned if failing to do so. Vitamin supplements may also be promoted and inappropriately used — other than Vitamin C which may be prescribed as an organic acid to reduce the urinary pH to enhance the actions of methenamine.

It is also worth emphasising that sedative medication and opiates are not at all appropriate because they induce dependency without contributing to treatment. Appropriate analgesia will be addressed in a later chapter.

Snake oil merchants

There is a pattern to spot. A basic scientific phenomenon is adopted, for example, interference with *Escherichia coli* adhesion molecules or GAG on urothelial cells. Laboratory studies that show some agent altering these functions are identified. A story about the pathophysiological mechanisms of the disease that co-opts these properties is invented. A medication is proposed containing a chemical that sounds like it might influence the imagined pathophysiology. Another story about how this medication works is created. These tales will contain some kernels of fact but abound with wishful thinking and preposterous extrapolation. The supporting evidence is invariably shoddy, sparse or "being written up". There may be papers from pseudo-scientific publications; beware they look so convincing [44]. These medications are usually ineffective, harmless and terribly expensive.

If you challenge those selling this rubbish, regardless of how assertive you are about the science and the holes in their claims, these salesmen prove weirdly impassive, unmoved by the criticisms of their claims. Some patient support organisations are sponsored by these merchants or they sell these products themselves or oblige with paid endorsements. The sales companies will commission qualified doctors, suitably clad in scrubs with stethoscope across the shoulders, to recommend their products using video that always feature a happy patient. It's kitsch, clichéd and the evidence is anecdotal; have these doctors no shame? The promotions are brimming with sophisticated financial conflicts of interest.

Marketing people play on our cognitive biases. Our intuitions drive us to want to believe congenial, charming people who flatter us. We are naturally repelled by those stroppy, arrogant, dissenters who challenge them. A video featuring a doctor in uniform or scrubs will convince; we trust them, not appreciating that they were remunerated. High-quality images and video animation persuade; gifts and hospitality serve a purpose. The system stinks and the patients pay.

So what to do about this? There is a simple option: you must ask for evidence of the therapeutic effect size. Forget p-values, R-values or what Professor *Giveusyarmoney* says: ask for the "clinical effect size"; demand an outcome measure, relevant and important to the patients. It is so important that we shall repeat the effect size calculation here:

Calculate the change in outcome measure during active treatment: the within active-group change:

$Change_{active}$ = [End study score active] − [Start study score active]

Calculate the same for the controls or placebo group.

The within control-group change:

$Change_{control}$ = [End study score control] − [Start study score control]

The effect size is the difference between the two.

Effect size = $Change_{active}$ − $Change_{control}$.

Note Change_active is not the effect size but the mountebanks will try to dupe you with Change_active and the associated p-value. Beware of the phrase "percentage of patients who improved" or other specious flannel.

Surgical interventions

The **urethral dilation** may have its roots in the symptoms associated with UTI. Voiding dysfunction including hesitancy, reduced stream, intermittency, terminal dribbling, post-micturition dribbling and double voiding are sensitive markers of infection in men and women [45]. They are often present because of infection, despite the absence of pain and may precede the pain whilst infection is building. It would seem that the inflammation and oedema of the urethra causes an obstruction to outflow and therefore a problem with voiding. Rarely, this can lead to acute retention. Unfortunately, the absence of pain can divert our attention from the true cause of the mischief. It is often assumed that residual urine left in the bladder because of voiding dysfunction is the cause of infection. Our evidence points to the opposite and that the infection causes the residual [46]. Some may think that this physiological obstruction could be alleviated by dilating the urethra, but that would be destructive; treating infection is a more conservative approach. A recent review concluded "There is no evidence supporting an appropriate role for urethral dilation in girls and women with recurrent UTI and dysfunctional voiding" [47].

Cystodistension seems to be justified by conjectured effects for which therapeutic claims are then imagined. It is another example of an intuition leaping from conception to action with zero scientific scrutiny on the way. There is no reason to expect that stretching the bladder will benefit cystitis or UTI, although the antibiotic administered during the procedure may be relevant [48, 49]. A recent systematic review commented: "The quality of available evidence falls below the level that would be expected of a new intervention". Ergo; the evidence is dismally appalling; this being emphasised by a concluding comment: "It is debatable whether cystodistension should be performed at all. However, pragmatically, given the lack of contemporaneous evidence, cystodistension may be utilised for the initial diagnosis of BPS only". There is a widespread assumption that mucosal bleeding, aka "glomerulations" after bladder distension, in the absence of macroscopic ulceration is diagnostic of IC/PBS/BPS [50], but this is not credible; innate immunity uses vascular dilation, capillary engorgement and increased permeability to deliver the inflammatory response. Stretching blood vessels in this situation is bound to cause them to bleed, just as we develop nosebleeds with winter cold viruses. Glomerulations may be signs of inflammation. It is cringingly silly to espy glomerulations and thus prescribe bladder instillations to repair the GAG layer; that is not practising medicine.

Fulguration

During fulguration an insulated electrode with a metal point is held against the bladder wall whilst a current is passed so that the point heats up and burns the tissues. It is used to treat tumours and prostate enlargement. It is advocated for interstitial cystitis and Hunner's ulcers but there are no proper clinical trials, just various anecdotal essays dressed up as these. We know that some use it to burn patches of metaplasia seen on the urothelial surface. We know little about the pathophysiology of macroscopic metaplasia; it is unstudied. It may differ from microscopic metaplasia, the innate immune response to infection. What is the scientific explanation of fulguration's action? In our context, the pathology would imply it to be futile.

We wonder whether it has crept in because of the politician's fallacy:

- We must do something.
- This is something.
- Therefore, we must do this.

Intermittent self-catheterisation

Much is made of residual urine in the bladder which is fingered as a cause of recurrent urinary infection. There is no evidence for this widely held belief. We shall describe later how voiding symptoms are sensitive markers of infection, presumably because inflammation and oedema obstructs the outflow tract. Infection may be correlated with voiding dysfunction because it is the cause. Some poor people are made to use intermittent self-catheterisation because they have a residual of over 150ml; again there is no justifying evidence. We tested the proposition in patients treated with botulinum toxin injections and intermittent self-catheterisation fell at the first rung by failing to correlate with changes in infection rates. Thus, as far as infection is concerned, intermittent catheterisation seems spurious and meddlesome [46].

Urovaccines

Before we discuss this, it is worth explaining a proper drug discovery programme:

- Characterisation of the pathophysiology of concern.
- Identification of drug targets.
- Screening for suitable pharmaceutical molecules.
- Characterisation of the chosen product(s).
- Pharmacokinetics and drug disposition.
- Preclinical toxicology testing.
- Bioanalytical testing.
- Proof of concept study.
- Clinical trials.

It is unacceptable to move from some idea into clinical prescription without achieving the scientific understanding that the above sequence will allow. It is equally deplorable to invent explanations for how an agent might achieve an imagined outcome and lay claim to these for your product. It is unforgiveable to fail to conduct the necessary clinical trials properly. Contentious clinicians should insist on these standards, otherwise their patients will pay through disappointment, adversity and impoverishment.

Uromune® is an immunomodulation therapy administered via a sublingual spray. It is composed of inactivated whole bacteria comprising the four most common uropathogenic organisms — *Escherichia coli*, *Klebsiella pneumoniae*, *Proteus vulgaris* and *Enterococcus faecalis*. It astonishes us that it is being used by clinicians to treat recurrent genitourinary infections; by what authority? Since when has a suspension of deactivated bacteria in a glycerinated medium, administered sublingually, influenced the immune function of the urinary tract? Where is the evidence of the immune activation and how does this therapy target the correct causative microbes? Causation is a major problem in understanding UTI.

The dominant pathology of cUTI is the parasitisation of the urothelial cells. It is evident that this process provokes an immune response. How on earth can the oral deactivated bacteria improve on the inoculation of the bladder by live bacteria?

This is the quality of the clinical research. A paper published in the *British Journal of Urology International* [51] reported on:

"77 women with culture-positive recurrent UTIs who were given a Uromune sublingual vaccine for a period of 3 months. Prospective observational follow-up was via a nurse phone consultation for up to 12 months. Symptoms of infections, when reported, were confirmed by the patients' GPs, with a urinary sample analysed for microscopy, culture and sensitivity prior to commencement of antibiotic therapy."

There were no controls and the outcome measure was a proven non-starter.

This underwhelming faux science was preceded by a retrospective case-note review of 669 women with recurrent UTI who were treated with Uromune® [52] and then followed by an equally, non-comparative, uncontrolled open study on 784 patients using the same hopelessly discredited outcome measure [53]. This science is as holed as a colander after a strafing but the promoters will argue their case vehemently using rhetorical sophistry. It makes a good paradigm illustrating these promotional methods.

Here is a quotation from just one urology clinic about Uromune®: "Cost for two 9ml spray dispensers which is sufficient for one 3/12 treatment regime is: $320.40 + delivery charge"; the patients have to pay for this.

Needless to say other manufacturers are jumping on this gravy train with their own versions of these urovaccines which exploit the vulnerable and put us to shame. It is not medicine to propose a treatment just in case it might work.

Do we administer orally, suspensions of deactivated bacteria to immunize against pneumonia, septicaemia or any other bacterial infection?

Memes and marketing

A meme, coined by Richard Dawkins in *The Selfish Gene* [54], is an idea that reproduces bypassing from one person's mind to another. Some memes are particularly powerful and parasitise our belief systems tenaciously. A successful meme continues to spread, exponentially through a social group. Good examples are found in the promotion of GAG layer replacement but similar meme infestations are ubiquitous. A company, marketing a quack remedy, will write a pseudoscientific explanation of the action, usually with diagrams, and distribute this on leaflets and labelling. Clinicians may read this and retain it, assuming it to be scientifically valid. When asked about the product they parrot this pseudoscience which is written to imply sagacious knowledge about mechanisms. Thus, a marketing blurb becomes a meme and infects colleagues and patients alike. Pseudoscientific, industry-created memes are reproduced in lectures, review papers, books and answers on social media. The patients have the "My doctor says" vector for spreading the infection. You do not have to prescribe to be a super-spreader. The advertisers know that most of us would prefer to answer with an apparently knowledgeable response instead of admitting to ignorance. Memes will promote remedies without evidence and despite the publication of falsifying data. Because they are such effective parasites, the host will defend them assertively with logical fallacies. We address a similar phenomenon of nature, later in the book.

Researchers may also generate false memes, particularly given their propensity to elaborate hypothetical explanations for their data as if proved. Because of the plethora of press viewpoint pieces we are desensitised to the blarney of opinions expressed as fact. Inappropriate rhetoric infests the parlance of science. Researchers describe their work using overwrought boastful clichés with big adjectives and utmost adverbs: totally novel, globally innovative, excellent, state-of-the-art, shifting paradigms, not to forget the hedge cutting too; how did that ever get in? It is embarrassing nonsense puffed with grandiloquent bombast. Listen to the quiet ones; they are so much more interesting.

Scamming

Max Frisch in 1953 wrote a play *The Fire Raisers*, a powerful story, worth seeing; it is available on YouTube. The main character, Biedermann, is convinced that he would never be taken in by scammers. Nevertheless, he invites into his house two apparent arsonists. They fill his loft with cans of petrol. Biedermann helps these intruders with their efforts to the extent of assisting in assembling a detonating fuse. He refuses to believe that these charming, gracious people are set on burning down his house, despite the evidence.

It is understandable that we are distraught and ashamed of ourselves when taken in by a financial scam. Being emailed or telephoned by scammers is unpleasant and causes upset. Nevertheless, we are indulgent of practices that are not much different. The sale of quack remedies and specious tests are burgeoning and promoted by clinicians, patients and through commercial stands at our conferences. It is like a Ponzi scheme with participants inveigling their friends and families to participate. The commitment generated can be so tenacious that the persuaded are affronted when the absence of evidence is pointed out.

Nowadays the internet enables a fact check to be secured inside a few minutes. We can search PubMed for free, thereby reading the scientific abstracts. There is no good reason for not being informed of an evidence dearth. To test this, search now and find a good reason for paying to have your bladder insufflated with ozone; you are better off bending over windward on the beach at Bognor.

Our Twitter account attracts many queries of the form "What do you think about this diet/remedy/test?" We have learned this to be an infinite, exhausting series that will never end; it is fed by the resourcefulness of the hawkers and lapped up by willing consumers. Nowadays we seek to simplify our response to a Socratic query; "So what evidence have you found to justify the question?" We all have responsibility for judging the efficacy of remedies, tests and interventions. Rightly, the existentialists insisted that we should take responsibility for our choices. There is no point in special pleading desperation, that does not right a wrong. We must retain control of those who seek to influence our lives and prevent them from exploiting our vulnerability. The scammers do not respect us; they think that we are suckers.

References

1. Hanno P, Lin A, Nordling J, et al. Bladder Pain Syndrome Committee of the International Consultation on Incontinence. Neurourol Urodyn 2010; 29(1): 191-8.

2. Hanno PM, Landis JR, Matthews-Cook Y, et al. The diagnosis of interstitial cystitis revisited: lessons learned from the National Institutes of Health Interstitial Cystitis Database study. J Urol 1999; 161(2): 553-7.

3. Warren JW, Meyer WA, Greenberg P, et al. Using the International Continence Society's definition of painful bladder syndrome. Urology 2006; 67(6): 1138-42.

4. Doyle AC. The case-book of Sherlock Holmes. Leipzig: Bernhard Tauchnitz; 1927.

5. Parsons CL. Bladder surface glycosaminoglycan: efficient mechanism of environmental adaptation. Urology 1986; 27(2 Suppl): 9-14.

6. Parsons CL, Hurst RE. Decreased urinary uronic acid levels in individuals with interstitial cystitis. J Urol 1990; 143(4): 690-3.

7. Nickel JC, Emerson L, Cornish J. The bladder mucus (glycosaminoglycan) layer in interstitial cystitis. J Urol 1993; 149(4): 716-8.

8. Parsons CL. A model for the function of glycosaminoglycans in the urinary tract. World J Urol 1994; 12(1): 38-42.

9. Erickson DR, Sheykhnazari M, Ordille S, et al. Increased urinary hyaluronic acid and interstitial cystitis. J Urol 1998; 160(4): 1282-4.

10. Bai X, Bame KJ, Habuchi H, et al. Turnover of heparan sulfate depends on 2-O-sulfation of uronic acids. J Biol Chem 1997; 272(37): 23172-9.

11. Yanagishita M, Hascall VC. Cell surface heparan sulfate proteoglycans. J Biol Chem 1992; 267(14): 9451-4.

12. Holm-Bentzen M, Jacobsen F, Nerstrom B, *et al.* A prospective double-blind clinically controlled multicenter trial of sodium pentosanpolysulfate in the treatment of interstitial cystitis and related painful bladder disease. *J Urol* 1987; 138(3): 503-7.

13. Fritjofsson A, Fall M, Juhlin R, *et al.* Treatment of ulcer and nonulcer interstitial cystitis with sodium pentosanpolysulfate: a multicenter trial. *J Urol* 1987; 138(3): 508-12.

14. Swamy S, Barcella W, De Iorio M, *et al.* Recalcitrant chronic bladder pain and recurrent cystitis but negative urinalysis: what should we do? *Int Urogynecol J* 2018; 29(7): 1035-43.

15. Swamy S, Kupelian AS, Khasriya R, *et al.* Cross-over data supporting long-term antibiotic treatment in patients with painful lower urinary tract symptoms, pyuria and negative urinalysis. *Int Urogynecol J* 2019; 30(3): 409-14.

16. Nickel JC, Herschorn S, Whitmore KE, *et al.* Pentosan polysulfate sodium for treatment of interstitial cystitis/bladder pain syndrome: insights from a randomized, double-blind, placebo controlled study. *J Urol* 2015; 193(3): 857-62.

17. Hanif AM, Armenti ST, Taylor SC, *et al.* Phenotypic spectrum of pentosan polysulfate sodium-associated maculopathy: a multicenter study. *JAMA Ophthalmol* 2019; 137(11): 1275-82.

18. Cervigni M, Sommariva M, Tenaglia R, *et al.* A randomized, open-label, multicenter study of the efficacy and safety of intravesical hyaluronic acid and chondroitin sulfate versus dimethyl sulfoxide in women with bladder pain syndrome/interstitial cystitis. *Neurourol Urodyn* 2017; 36(4): 1178-86.

19. Cicione A, Cantiello F, Ucciero G, *et al.* Restoring the glycosaminoglycans layer in recurrent cystitis: experimental and clinical foundations. *Int J Urol* 2014; 21(8): 763-8.

20. O'Leary MP, Sant GR, Fowler FJ, Jr., *et al.* The interstitial cystitis symptom index and problem index. *Urology* 1997; 49(5A Suppl): 58-63.

21. Lai MC, Kuo YC, Kuo HC. Intravesical hyaluronic acid for interstitial cystitis/painful bladder syndrome: a comparative randomized assessment of different regimens. *Int J Urol* 2013; 20(2): 203-7.

22. Bade JJ, Laseur M, Nieuwenburg A, *et al.* A placebo-controlled study of intravesical pentosanpolysulphate for the treatment of interstitial cystitis. *Br J Urol* 1997; 79(2): 168-71.

23. Morales A, Emerson L, Nickel JC. Intravesical hyaluronic acid in the treatment of refractory interstitial cystitis. *Urology* 1997; 49(5A Suppl): 111-3.

24. Davis EL, El Khoudary SR, Talbott EO, *et al.* Safety and efficacy of the use of intravesical and oral pentosan polysulfate sodium for interstitial cystitis: a randomized double-blind clinical trial. *J Urol* 2008; 179(1): 177-85.

25. Nickel JC, Egerdie B, Downey J, *et al.* A real-life multicentre clinical practice study to evaluate the efficacy and safety of intravesical chondroitin sulphate for the treatment of interstitial cystitis. *BJU Int* 2009; 103(1): 56-60.

26. Daha LK, Riedl CR, Lazar D, *et al.* Effect of intravesical glycosaminoglycan substitution therapy on bladder pain syndrome/interstitial cystitis, bladder capacity and potassium sensitivity. *Scand J Urol Nephrol* 2008; 42(4): 369-72.

27. Nickel JC, Egerdie RB, Steinhoff G, *et al.* A multicenter, randomized, double-blind, parallel group pilot evaluation of the efficacy and safety of intravesical sodium chondroitin sulfate versus vehicle control in patients with interstitial cystitis/painful bladder syndrome. *Urology* 2010; 76(4): 804-9.

28. Lv YS, Zhou HL, Mao HP, *et al.* Intravesical hyaluronic acid and alkalinized lidocaine for the treatment of severe painful bladder syndrome/interstitial cystitis. *Int Urogynecol J* 2012; 23(12): 1715-20.

29. Pyo JS, Cho WJ. Systematic review and meta-analysis of intravesical hyaluronic acid and hyaluronic acid/chondroitin sulfate instillation for interstitial cystitis/painful bladder syndrome. *Cell Physiol Biochem* 2016; 39(4): 1618-25.

30. Zhang W, Deng X, Liu C, Wang X. Intravesical treatment for interstitial cystitis/painful bladder syndrome: a network meta-analysis. *Int Urogynecol J* 2017; 28(4): 515-25.

31. Barua JM, Arance I, Angulo JC, Riedl CR. A systematic review and meta-analysis on the efficacy of intravesical therapy for bladder pain syndrome/interstitial cystitis. *Int Urogynecol J* 2016; 27(8): 1137-47.

32. Dawson TE, Jamison J. Intravesical treatments for painful bladder syndrome/interstitial cystitis. *Cochrane Database Syst Rev* 2007; 4: CD006113.

33. Leitner L, Ujmajuridze A, Chanishvili N, *et al.* Intravesical bacteriophages for treating urinary tract infections in patients undergoing transurethral resection of the prostate: a randomised, placebo-controlled, double-blind clinical trial. *Lancet Infect Dis* 2020; doi: 10.1016/S1473-3099(20)30330-3.

34. Blatherwick NR, Long ML. Studies of urinary tract acidity. II. The increased acidity produced by eating prunes and cranberries. *J Biol Chem* 1923; 57: 3.

35. Bodel PT, Cotran R, Kass EH. Cranberry juice and the antibacterial action of hippuric acid. *J Lab Clin Med* 1959; 54: 881-8.

36. Sobota AE. Inhibition of bacterial adherence by cranberry juice: potential use for the treatment of urinary tract infections. *J Urol* 1984; 131(5): 1013-6.

37. Juthani-Mehta M, Van Ness PH, Bianco L, *et al.* Effect of cranberry capsules on bacteriuria plus pyuria among older women in nursing homes: a randomized clinical trial. *JAMA* 2016; 316(18): 1879-87.

38.   Gupta A, Dwivedi M, Mahdi AA, *et al*. Inhibition of adherence of multi-drug resistant *E. coli* by proanthocyanidin. *Urol Res* 2012; 40(2): 143-50.

39.   Manach C, Williamson G, Morand C, *et al*. Bioavailability and bioefficacy of polyphenols in humans. I. Review of 97 bioavailability studies. *Am J Clin Nutr* 2005; 81(1 Suppl): 230s-42s.

40.   Genovese C, Davinelli S, Mangano K, *et al*. Effects of a new combination of plant extracts plus d-mannose for the management of uncomplicated recurrent urinary tract infections. *J Chemother* 2018; 30(2): 107-14.

41.   Mehta I, Zimmern P, Reitzer L. Enzymatic assay of d-mannose from urine. *Bioanalysis* 2018; 10(23): 1947-54.

42.   Kranjcec B, Papes D, Altarac S. D-mannose powder for prophylaxis of recurrent urinary tract infections in women: a randomized clinical trial. *World J Urol* 2014; 32(1): 79-84.

43.   Anderson GG, Palermo JJ, Schilling JD, *et al*. Intracellular bacterial biofilm-like pods in urinary tract infections. *Science* 2003; 301(5629): 105-7.

44.   Cukier S, Lalu M, Bryson GL, *et al*. Defining predatory journals and responding to the threat they pose: a modified Delphi consensus process. *BMJ* 2020; 10(2): e035561.

45.   Khasriya R, Barcella W, De Iorio M, *et al*. Lower urinary tract symptoms that predict microscopic pyuria. *Int Urogynecol J* 2018; 29(7): 1019-28.

46.   Collins L, Sathiananthamoorthy S, Fader M, Malone-Lee J. Intermittent catheterisation after botulinum toxin injections: the time to reassess our practice. *Int Urogynecol J* 2017; 28(9): 1351-6.

47.   Bazi T, Abou-Ghannam G, Khauli R. Female urethral dilation. *Int Urogynecol J* 2013; 24(9): 1435-44.

48.   Carey MM, Zreik A, Fenn NJ, *et al*. Should we use antibiotic prophylaxis for flexible cystoscopy? A systematic review and meta-analysis. *Urol Int* 2015; 95(3): 249-59.

49.   Zeng S, Zhang Z, Bai Y, *et al*. Antimicrobial agents for preventing urinary tract infections in adults undergoing cystoscopy. *Cochrane Database Syst Rev* 2019; 2: CD012305.

50.   Homma Y, Ueda T, Tomoe H, *et al*. Clinical guidelines for interstitial cystitis and hypersensitive bladder updated in 2015. *Int J Urol* 2016; 23(7): 542-9.

51.   Yang B, Foley S. First experience in the UK of treating women with recurrent urinary tract infections with the bacterial vaccine Uromune®. *BJU Int* 2018; 121(2): 289-92.

52.   Lorenzo-Gomez MF, Padilla-Fernandez B, Garcia-Cenador MB, *et al*. Comparison of sublingual therapeutic vaccine with antibiotics for the prophylaxis of recurrent urinary tract infections. *Front Cell Infect Microbiol* 2015; 5: 50.

53.   Ramirez Sevilla C, Gomez Lanza E, Manzanera JL, *et al*. Active immunoprophyilaxis with Uromune® decreases the recurrence of urinary tract infections at three and six months after treatment without relevant secondary effects. *BMC Infect Dis* 2019; 19(1): 901.

54.   Dawkins R. *The selfish gene*. Oxford: Oxford University Press; 1976.

Chapter 5

UTI and the testing mayhem

We do admit that we are approaching cystitis in an unusual order, but for good reason. UTI is bedevilled by many misunderstandings particularly diagnostic testing strategies. It seems best to clear these minefields before moving into the pathophysiology, assessment and treatment.

Prior to covering some investigations, it might help to recap on test functions, discussed in Chapter 2, ▓ Figure 2.1. We take a history and perform an examination, assimilating these data through induction. Next, we use imagination to conjecture an explanation for the evidence we gathered thereby abducting a hypothesis. This is speculative, so we deploy an error trap: we deduce a prediction, a consequence if the hypothesis be true. A test is used to check that prediction and thereby verify or falsify the hypothesis. This test must be validated for purpose and its limitations understood.

Beware of correlations

Tyler Vigen, who was born in 1991 in the USA, is a juris doctor graduate of Harvard Law School and a mathematician. Whilst he was a student he created the "Spurious correlations" website (https://tylervigen.com/spurious-correlations) where he provides graphs of amazing correlations that you may find seductive. In Charles Dickens' *A Christmas Carol*, Ebenezer Scrooge, experiencing ghostly nocturnal visitations, blamed his nightmares on eating a "crumb of cheese". This myth has persisted. Thus, if eating cheese is a cause of nightmares, we should expect a correlation between cheese consumption and death by tangling in bedsheets; "tangulation". Thus, we present data provided by Tyler Vigen (Figure 5.1), plotting the years 2000 to 2009 on the abscissa (x-axis) with the USA annual consumption of cheese and the number of deaths by tangulation on the ordinates (y-axes) (R=0.97, p<.0000000!). Perhaps Mr Scrooge was correct. Such correlations are spurious, but reflect non-random shared associations with undeclared confounders; in the example it is progress of time. Correlation is a statistical measure; substantive meaning hangs on the assumptions and hypothesis motivating the analysis; tangulation is not a plausible option.

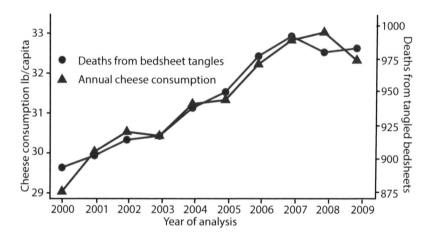

Figure 5.1. Deaths from tangled bedsheets and cheese consumption.

Hypothesis-free data searching may find group differences or correlations which are then promoted for test roles without sufficient diligence in seeking confounding explanatory causes. For example, many urodynamic measures are explained by the physics of bladder capacity differences. An illustrative version of this type of analysis relevant to medicine was discussed in *The New England Journal of Medicine* by Messerli *et al* where chocolate consumption and cognitive function were linked to success in achieving Nobel prizes [1].

The urine culture

A MSU culture should not be the first test used but it has been granted the status of a powerful reference standard, so we must address this now, to provide context to what follows.

To a great extent, all over the world the diagnosis of UTI is predicated on a quantitative microbial culture applied to a clean catch midstream urine sample (MSU). The diagnostic threshold recommended is inconsistent varying between 10^2 and 10^6 colony forming units (cfu)/ml, of a single species of a known urinary pathogen. The source of these criteria is a paper by Kass in 1957. This reported a study of 74 women, with acute pyelonephritis, and 335 asymptomatic controls [2]. Subsequently, Kass used a sample of pregnant women with pyelonephritis to represent severe infection in a further analysis, during his quest for a diagnostic threshold which he set at 10^5 cfu/ml [3]. It is baffling that the 10^5 cfu/ml should have gone on to become the gold standard reference and gatekeeper to the diagnosis of UTI. Some did question the wisdom for this approach but their reflective views were ignored [4, 5]. The consequences have been calamitous.

Kass was wrong in assuming that the normal urinary tract was sterile; there was never any evidence for this. The corollary was to believe that a microbe, isolated from an uncontaminated specimen, must be a causative pathogen. The notion of a sterile normal bladder does not fit comfortably with Darwinian evolution, which expects colonisation of all niches, no matter how hostile [6]. Nowadays this presumption about the healthy bladder has been refuted [7-9]. The situation was further complicated because Koch's postulates have not been adapted in the light of contemporary knowledge. Koch insisted on a single species and so today we talk of "mixed growth of doubtful significance"; but we have come to recognise a polymicrobial urinary microbiome in health and disease with a considerable overlap [7-9].

Figure 5.2 comes from Kiren Gill's 2018 cohort study [10] of monthly comparative observations over a year. The data were obtained from spun sediment cultures [8]. It demonstrates the fact of a non-sterile normal bladder and the qualitative similarities in the bacteria that are colonising patients and controls.

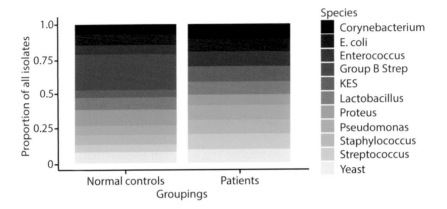

Figure 5.2. A comparison of species from spun sediment cultures, obtained from patients and controls.

This figure compares the species dispersion from urinary sediment cultures obtained from patients and controls over 12 months of observation (Gill et al) [10]. *There is substantial overlap without clear distinction. It is impossible to identify causation in such a situation. KES = Klebsiella spp., Enterobacter spp. and Serratia spp.*

Figure 5.3 comes from the same study. For each genus isolated from the cultures, the relative proportions expressed in patients and controls are compared and sorted to illustrate the differences and the overlap.

Figure 5.4 illustrates the culture methods that were used and compares the spun sediment culture to the standard 1µl inoculation of the culture agar which nowadays is chromogenic agar.

If the microbiome is polymicrobial and the microbial species show so much overlap with normal controls, we are in no position to attribute causation to our isolate which may well be a ubiquitous, easy to grow harmless mutualist, despite its reputation.

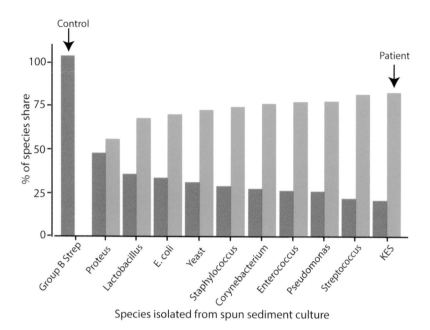

Species isolated from spun sediment culture

Figure 5.3. How the patients and controls share species between them.

This figure demonstrates how individual species are apportioned between patients and controls. Each column pair sums to 100%. The groups differ in how the species are distributed between them but there is much overlap. The difficulty in attributing disease causation is evident. The data are from Gill et al [10]. KES = Klebsiella spp., Enterobacter spp. and Serratia spp.

There is no evidence that abundance implies causation although this fallacy is being recycled to defend urinary DNA analysis. The truth is more complicated than such glib assumptions. The difference between patients and controls lies in the greater plethora of species in patients but there is so much overlap that it is impossible to identify the causative microbe(s) or distinguish infection from no infection on a culture result [7, 10]. Enhanced cultivation methods such as spun sediment cultures or broth cultures [8, 11] may well isolate many more microbial species than usual MSU cultures, but it is wrong to assume these bacteria are causal pathogens.

The discovery of the extensive bladder microbiome in health [8] means that we should revisit the term "asymptomatic bacteriuria". Normal people

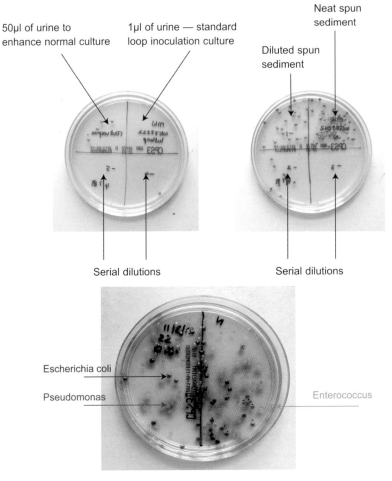

50µl of urine to
enhance normal culture

1µl of urine — standard
loop inoculation culture

Neat spun
sediment

Diluted spun
sediment

Serial dilutions

Serial dilutions

Escherichia coli

Pseudomonas

Enterococcus

The dyes in the chromogenic agar are used
to help identify the genus of the microbe

Figure 5.4. A comparison of culture methods: the spun sediment culture compared with standard inoculation of culture agar.

This figure illustrates the different approaches to culture using chromogenic agar. The standard hospital MSU culture uses a 1µl loop inoculation of the media with urine. We also tested a 50µl pipette inoculation which resulted in more isolates. Similarly, the spun sediment culture enhanced the delivery of isolates. Similar effects are achieved by dropping the diagnostic threshold to 10^3 cfu/ml. In all cases we can report richer results but none say anything about causation. Just because a bug is there it does not mean that it caused the disease.

without symptoms should have bacteria in the urine and these may show up in culture. Asymptomatic bacteriuria is a vestigial term that makes little sense today. Much is made of not treating it; why would you treat if the patients have no symptoms? You would risk killing harmless, probably beneficial mutualists.

Mixed growth of considerable significance

It is a common occurrence for patients to describe presenting to a doctor with typical symptoms of UTI and with urinalysis showing pyuria. However, they are not prescribed treatment with antibiotics because the MSU culture report comes back as "Mixed growth of doubtful significance".

Figure 5.5 depicts data that should rattle our confidence in the reassurance of mixed growth cultures. The data are from our monitoring activity and we plot the mean $\log_{10}$ pyuria counts with 95% confidence intervals on the ordinate (y-axis) for normal controls, and those groups with negative culture, mixed growth and positive culture. There is something wrong with the negative culture patients but seriously so with the mixed growth group.

We should not be surprised by this result. The assessment of mixed growth cultures is based on assumptions that have been refuted. The voices proclaiming infection are the symptoms, signs and pyuria [12]. It is not right to dismiss a UTI diagnosis because of a mixed growth culture.

We have to accept this; the MSU culture and enhanced alternatives [8] are incapable of arbitrating UTI or no UTI. Cultures are also unable to identify the causative microbe(s) and so their antimicrobial sensitivity data may be misleading. In a later chapter we shall present evidence that sensitivity data from cultures encourage the use of needlessly broad-spectrum antibiotics.

It is flatly wrong to inform patients, with relevant symptoms, that they could not have an infection because the urine cultures were negative or showed a mixed culture.

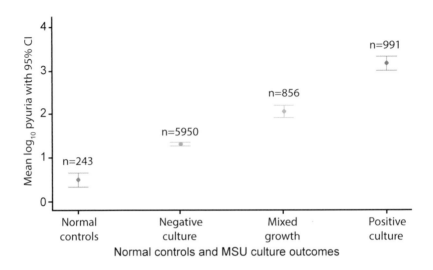

Figure 5.5. Patients with lower urinary tract symptoms (LUTS) mean log pyuria and 95% CI across culture results.

The data in this figure show how LUTS patients with negative cultures may nevertheless demonstrate pyuria which is not normal and the most likely explanation is infection. The mixed growth culture group are also notably abnormal. As an aside, these are 95% confidence intervals and so there is no need to quote the p-values since it is self-evident that p<.05 and after that we are only interested in the sizes of the between group differences, i.e. the effect sizes.

Genomics

16S rRNA shotgun metagenomics urinalysis is the same as "next generation sequencing" (NGS). It is a useful research tool but not an option in the clinical situation at this time. It is mistakenly promoted by clinicians and patients' advocacy websites as an appropriate diagnostic tool, but that does not bear scrutiny. These methods are great for detecting what there is but they say nothing about causation [7]. The signals that identify the presence of microbial genes use the polymerase chain reaction (PCR) to amplify the genetic code massively so the insignificant is given a loud voice.

A while ago we were perplexed by an aberrant signal in our control channel for microbial NGS PCR analysis of urine. Chancing the fundamental attribution error, we besmirched the PhD student alleging dirty habits. After we had been told to grow up, the amazingly, ultra-hygienic, fragrant postgraduate sequenced *Halomonas spp.* in the control. The DNA polymerase we used was a modified enzyme isolated from a strain of *Pyrococcus spp.* that inhabits deep-sea hydrothermal vents. A species of *Halomonas* shares that habitat. In short, we had amplified a miniscule deep ocean contamination of the polymerase. The moral? Do not defame the postgrads; you will be abased, and watch what you claim about NGS PCR fingering the cause.

It is a wild leap to promote NGS as useful, informative testing for clinical management. Nevertheless, there are companies who sell their NGS services for cystitis without explaining how the data should inform treatment.

Using NGS we and others found that controls exhibit approaching 600 species, with patients about 2% more. There is considerable overlap (85%) which is well shown in Figure 5.6 where we compare the number of different species found in patients and normal controls [7, 9]. Figure 5.7 addresses the same data but presents the relative proportion of the most numerous 20 species isolated from the same groups. Patients have greater species dispersion but that does not incriminate the causative organisms. Some assert that relative abundance indicates causation although published data contradict that [7]. There is enthusiasm for the DNA methods identifying antimicrobial resistance genes. This is important but not useful therapeutically if causation is unattributed.

If companies seek to market expensive NGS testing or enhanced cultures for UTI they should answer the following questions in their promotional literature:

- Do you identify disease cause?
- Should your resistance data guide antibiotic choice?
- How should doctors use your data?
- What is your evidence for 1 to 3?

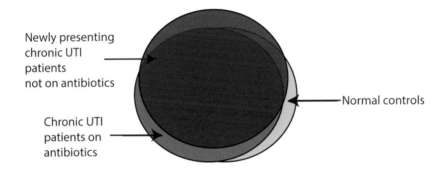

Figure 5.6. A three-way Venn diagram demonstrating the overlap in species identified in the urine by 16S rRNA ribotyping. The comparison is between normal controls, patients with untreated UTI and patients taking antibiotics for UTI.

In this analysis we identified approximately 590 species in patients presenting new with symptoms of cUTI, 600 in patients on treatment for cUTI and 580 in normal controls. There was a 500 species overlap between all three groups. This represents a 2% difference in species with an 85% overlap. It would be preposterous to claim that these differences offered diagnostic discrimination or evidence of causation. Data from Sathiananthamoorthy et al [7].

If they will not answer, it would suggest that a red flag has been raised. Medicine boasts a history of enthusiasm for methods based on false assumptions about causation [13]. Making unsubstantiated claims for NGS is to repeat the mistakes of the past; the MSU culture was not validated for causation and the patients paid a terrible price. Given the lesson of such unnecessary suffering, we must not repeat this folly. Macbeth, the Thane of Glamis and Cawdor, put it beautifully: "All our yesterdays have lighted fools the way to dusty death" (Macbeth act 5, scene 5).

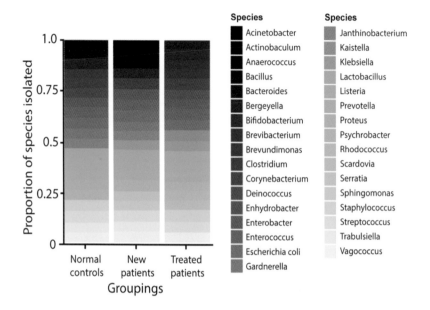

Figure 5.7. The top 20 species from 16S rRNA ribotyping.

In this analysis we drew the top 20 most abundant species isolated from normal controls, untreated patients and patients being treated with antibiotics. Once we start using 16S rRNA ribotyping the relative proportions tend to be similar. There are differences but they are unhelpful in addressing the problem of causation.

The genomic probe-based pocket tests are the latest craze. They too are based on false assumptions. Grandiloquent claims are made for the capabilities for point-of-care (lingo = "POC") tests that are claimed to identify the offending microbe: "Imagine, knowing the microbial cause of the UTI within minutes, in your consulting room?" might be captivating but it is mistaken, the method speeding the commission of the errors of the past. No, we can't imagine. There is no justification for such attributions. Without resolution of causation these microbial identification methods are just expensive dream-wares.

Report a scientific discovery contrasting patients and controls and some clinicians immediately propose test applications. A method may be suited to laboratory study of the disease but is inappropriate for clinical work. Measurement differences rarely invite legitimate test applications. In any case, difference is not the same as distinction; test strategies often confuse those two and waste life trying to force the test to fit the disease phenotype.

The dipstick tests for leucocyte esterase and nitrite

The news gets worse; the surrogate methods of testing for UTI are calibrated to MSU culture using the Kass criteria of 10^5 cfu/ml; the reference standard that is hopelessly discredited. It is inevitable that these tests should prove to be unsound too.

The dipsticks were launched onto the markets and into our guidelines without rigorous validation. In recent years we have submitted them to the scrutiny that should have preceded their introduction and they have performed exceedingly badly [7, 10, 14, 15]. They are insensitive and alarmingly unreliable.

One of the properties of the leucocyte esterase test is the high specificity so that if positive, be assured that there is a pyuria and probably in abundance. Given symptoms and a positive result the diagnosis of UTI is almost certain; a negative result says nothing. If there are no symptoms with a positive test, treatment is not indicated since the innate immunity would seem to be coping. The leucocyte esterase test says nothing about bacteriuria, only pyuria. The nitrite test says nothing of any use.

There is no justification for using leucocyte esterase and nitrite dipsticks to exclude the UTI diagnosis.

Dipsticks for other markers

Dipstick analysis is one of the simple and readily available tests and it is sensible to understand what the different signals may or may not convey.

Blood on dipsticks

The dipsticks are sensitive to blood so a positive result should not be acted on without microscopic confirmation of the reaction; it is unfair on the patient to act otherwise. Guidelines vary but the threshold for concern is often stated as >3 rbc per high powered field (hpf = x40 objective/equivalent to about 20 rbc/µl) [16]. You may have significant haematuria without proteinuria.

UTI, which causes dysuria, generates an inflammatory reaction with dilated mucosal blood vessels which are friable and may bleed, thus haematuria is a recognised manifestation of UTI. Haematuria, particularly frank haematuria, is a key marker of bladder cancer. Be aware that dysuria may also be present. So, if we find haematuria in someone with symptoms of UTI should we arrange urine cytology, renal tract imaging, and flexible cystoscopy? We do not want to cystoscope an infected bladder unnecessarily but cUTI takes a long time to clear.

Frank haematuria should be investigated. Microscopic haematuria should first be investigated based on consideration of the risk factors; male gender, persons aged ≥35 years, a history of smoking, occupational carcinogen exposure, and unexplained recalcitrant dysuria when aged ≥60. If haematuria persists we investigate regardless. We should not overlook women with risk factors [17, 18]. There is no evidence for routine cystoscopies in patients presenting with symptoms of cUTI or IC/BPS/PBS.

Protein

The glomerular capillaries and the lattice-like glomerular basement membrane have holes large enough to let albumin and small protein molecules, which are negatively charged, through into the urine. A functioning glomerular cell places anionic, negatively charged, proteoglycan molecules (aka GAG) on the basement membrane lattice. These repel the negatively charged proteins so that they do not pass through into the urine. If the glomerular cells sicken this process is compromised and albumin and protein leaks into the urine [19]. Thus, proteinuria (albuminuria) is a marker of glomerular disease and points to the kidney where diabetes and hypertension are the main suspects. Whatever the cause it merits conscientious assessment. The dipsticks are sensitive and may give false positives. It is easy enough to check the significance of dipstick detected proteinuria by sending the sample for a protein:creatinine ratio analysis [20].

Proteinuria is no marker of infection and should not be explained away by infection or used to diagnose it.

The glomeruli are highly vascular structures that will bleed readily. Thus, if the glomeruli are being damaged, as by glomerulonephritis, we should expect to find blood in the urine. Blood and protein in the urine is indicative of glomerulonephritis and may represent an acute nephrological emergency if a crescentic nephritis is the culprit. We should not sit on unexplained haematuria and proteinuria [21].

Glucose

There should not be glucose in the urine. It is a sign of diabetes to be dealt with appropriately. Untreated diabetes will compromise the ability of a patient to cope with a UTI so it is relevant to care. If a patient has presented with a history, symptoms and signs of UTI we should not be tempted to attribute them to glycosuria. That is only feasible if there is no microscopic pyuria; negative dipstick pyuria is not good enough.

Ketones

Ketones appear in the urine when the body is breaking down fat and the usual cause is fasting of some kind. If ketones co-exist with glucose, that is a potentially serious matter and the patient's diabetes needs to be addressed urgently and a urine infection treated promptly.

pH

The pH of the urine is of no help in the assessment of UTI. This has been examined exhaustively and various popular theories, particularly on causative bacterial species, have not stood up to scrutiny.

Specific gravity

This can be useful. If 1.000 we ask whether the patient is drinking too much fluid. People in fear of UTI may do this and it is not a wise option to follow. If it is over 1.015 we ask about the use of fluid restriction and reasons for doing this.

Bilirubin

For bilirubin to be in the urine there has to be an obstructive jaundice which may be extrahepatic due to a stone or tumour or intrahepatic as with hepatitis.

Urobilinogen

If there is bilirubin but no urobilinogen, we are probably looking at an extrahepatic obstruction and the patient requires a suitable ultrasound scan. If there is bilirubin and urobilinogen is increased, we are probably looking at a hepatitis.

Renal tract ultrasound scan

If someone has a chronic UTI (cUTI), renal tract ultrasound is necessary to seek out anatomical abnormalities and stones [22]. Whilst it is excellent at identifying a voiding problem that may not be relevant, residual urine may have no causative role in UTI [23]. Bladder wall thickness was once of interest in our field but disappointingly this waned when found not to correlate with urodynamic findings [24]. We might expect diffuse bladder wall thickening to occur with chronic cystitis because of urothelial hyperplasia or it may reflect detrusor hypertrophy associated with the overactive bladder. Focal bladder wall thickness should alert us to the possibility of a tumour of some kind. In our clinical practice we are conscious of reports of mild slight upper tract dilation in our cUTI patients [25]. It would be a service to us all if some curious clinicians would conduct some studies to clarify the significance of bladder wall thickness and upper tract dilation associated with cUTI.

If someone is overweight (BMI >30) an ultrasound scan may not be informative. It is then necessary to consider whether the radiation exposure of a CT scan is reasonable.

CT scan

A CT scan involves a radiation dose and should not be advocated lightly. There is no justification for routine CT scans in the assessment of cUTI. There has to be a coherent hypothesis for the scan to test before requesting this imaging [26].

The CT scan is sometimes justified on its greater sensitivity and specificity in detecting renal stones but this has not stood up to scrutiny in a RCT [27].

MRI scan

There are no validated indications for the routine use of MRI scanning in the assessment of UTI [28].

Urodynamic studies

The urodynamic study has no place in the assessment of a person troubled by urinary tract infections. The test should not be conducted anyway in someone with pyuria. Unfortunately, these principles are not realised in clinical practice.

This test has an interesting illustrative history. It was first used to assess women presenting with urinary incontinence. It was noticed that bladder contractions were seen in some patients during bladder filling. These were attributed a pathological status termed "detrusor instability" [29]. A standing coughing stress test was included in the protocol and used to diagnose stress incontinence [30]. The relationship between the voiding flow rate and the detrusor pressure was claimed to measure outflow obstruction [31]. Further finessing described a flaccid bladder and a stiff bladder, lacking compliance. Diagnostic categorisation with demarcation thresholds were adopted. Eventually, test guidelines were developed but without a coherent explanation of the related pathology [32].

The validation of urodynamics never included external references to independent measures of pathophysiology. Instead it self-referenced, self-validated and was justified by circular reasoning. Advocates argued the case by starting with urodynamics as a premise, but their inference has led back to urodynamics as the conclusion. If seeking to argue the case for urodynamics, it is not appropriate to include the test in the premise. It worked like this: the urodynamics showed some change. The clinician sought out a clinical phenotype that complemented this. The "subjective" phenotype was redefined *post hoc* in terms of the "objective" urodynamics. The test found meaning only in ideological presumptions about objectivity with appeals to self-evident truth. It still floats independently in the ether, unfettered by connections to anything else. The logic is an example of question begging, albeit in seductive form. When comparative studies of the urodynamic categories and clinical phenotype have been achieved, between group differences in urodynamic measures are evident, but dispersion and overlapping variances preclude discrimination. If a diagnostic test cannot discriminate it is not useful.

The categorisation of the symptomatic phenotype as subjective and urodynamics objective, reflects an inexplicable scepticism about the patients' symptoms. This was crystallised in the slogan "The bladder is an unreliable witness" [33], drawing on the evidence-free conviction that urodynamics is an observer superior to symptoms. Who says a patient cannot describe her experience? Why shouldn't the test be wrong? The scientific evidence implies this, but woe unto you if you say so.

Randomised trials applied to urodynamics have failed to demonstrate clinical efficacy for assessing the overactive bladder [34]. In that study symptomatic patients without detrusor instability responded to treatment identically to patients with the urodynamic finding. A RCT of urodynamics for female stress incontinence [35] refuted all assumptions about the test, which proved redundant to management. Finally, the theoretical principles for assessing outflow obstruction did not stand up to clinical scrutiny [36].

The urodynamic test, along with the cystoscopy, plays a role in providing an escape diversion when a clinician is confounded. Do not know what to do? Book one of these tests and move onto the next patient. The fundamental response to that is why? "What is the hypothesis that you plan to test with this intrusive and invasive investigation? On what evidence is the hypothesis based?"

Cystoscopy

The use of cystoscopy is another perplexing matter. Haematuria is an indisputable indication for seeking out a bladder cancer. After that the recommendations are not consistent [37].

The other use of cystoscopy in this context is in the assessment of patients being considered for IC/PBS/BPS; a cystoscopy with hydrodistension of the bladder may be used to identify glomerulations, ulceration may be seen, and biopsies may exhibit the various features of chronic inflammation. To date, such findings have been interpreted on the understanding the infection has been excluded by urine culture but urine culture is not competent to do this.

Glomerulations are capillary bleeds resulting from damage to the bladder urothelium by stretching. Bloated capillaries rupture easily [38]. If the bladder is inflamed, a manifestation of vasodilation, we should expect glomerulations. Comparative studies have refuted the diagnostic relevance of glomerulations [39].

It is also claimed that the cystoscopy should be used to identify Hunner's ulcers on the assumption that these are specific to IC. However, the histology of Hunner's ulcers is a non-specific chronic inflammation with urothelial ulceration [40], but the histology of chronic cystitis is that of a non-specific chronic inflammatory reaction with some urothelial ulceration [41]. The much-vaunted notion that mast cell infiltration has specificity is also debunked [42, 43].

The literature on the pathology of IC/PBS/BPS is full of contradictory claims. It seems to describe heroic efforts to force symptoms and signs to make sense without infection when these are wholly compatible with infection. The incompetence of the urine culture may be a clue to the explanation.

Inflammatory markers

The systemic markers of inflammation, ESR and CRP, have no role in the assessment of UTI. They may be affected if the infection spills over into the circulation. It is possible to have pyelonephritis without these being elevated [44, 45]. Such measures are not necessary anyway since the symptoms and signs say it all. It is quite wrong to believe that normal values exclude UTI.

Floundering over causation

The tests criticised in this chapter are frequently justified on the evidence of between group quantitative differences in measures. If you count more colonies of a species in your patients, compared to controls, it is tempting to attribute a causative role to the abundant microbe, but it is not correct. The statistical test used to compare groups for significant differences is the analysis of variance (ANOVA). It is not widely appreciated that the ANOVA calculations are the same as the linear regression calculations, which are used to measure correlation. They are the same analysis. We know that the cock crow does not cause the sun to rise but they surely correlate. We assume that we are too sophisticated to make such rudimentary attribution errors. However, it is true that today, clinicians, using enhanced cultures or 16S rRNA ribotyping, are attributing causation on the evidence of abundance, thereby confusing correlation with causation without realising it. In a later chapter we shall explain why plentiful microbes may be innocent. Would that causation were as easy to resolve as implied; in truth it is a fiendishly difficult problem. We are too preoccupied with landing a tidy quick fix when the biology is not going to cooperate. We must be assiduous in considering the whole story, not just what suits our purpose. The USA presidential elections of 2020 provide an excellent, germane metaphor: Do not forget about the votes in the mail and count them.

References

1. Messerli FH. Chocolate consumption, cognitive function, and Nobel laureates. *N Engl J Med* 2012; 367(16): 1562-4.

2. Kass EH. Bacteriuria and the diagnosis of infection in the urinary tract. *Arch Intern Med* 1957; 100: 709-14.

3. Kass EH. Bacteriuria and pyelonephritis of pregnancy. *Arch Intern Med* 1960; 105: 194-8.

4. Stamm WE, Counts GW, Running KR, *et al*. Diagnosis of coliform infection in acutely dysuric women. *N Engl J Med* 1982; 307(8): 463-8.

5. Wear JB, Jr. Correlation of pyuria, stained urine smear, urine culture and the uroscreen test. *J Urol* 1966; 96(5): 808-11.

6. Adam PS, Borrel G, Brochier-Armanet C, Gribaldo S. The growing tree of Archaea: new perspectives on their diversity, evolution and ecology. *ISME J* 2017; 11(11): 2407-25.

7. Sathiananthamoorthy S, Malone-Lee J, Gill K, *et al*. Reassessment of routine midstream culture in diagnosis of urinary tract infection. *J Clin Microbiol* 2019; 57(3): 01452-18.

8. Khasriya R, Sathiananthamoorthy S, Ismail S, *et al*. Spectrum of bacterial colonization associated with urothelial cells from patients with chronic lower urinary tract symptoms. *J Clin Microbiol* 2013; 51(7): 2054-62.

9. Pearce MM, Hilt EE, Rosenfeld AB, *et al*. The female urinary microbiome: a comparison of women with and without urgency urinary incontinence. *mBio* 2014; 5(4): e01283-14.

10. Gill K, Kang R, Sathiananthamoorthy S, *et al*. A blinded observational cohort study of the microbiological ecology associated with pyuria and overactive bladder symptoms. *Int Urogynecol J* 2018; 29(10): 1493-500.

11. Aydogan TB, Gurpinar O, Eser OK, *et al*. A new look at the etiology of interstitial cystitis/bladder pain syndrome: extraordinary cultivations. *Int Urol Nephrol* 2019; 51(11): 1961-7.

12. Khasriya R, Barcella W, De Iorio M, *et al*. Lower urinary tract symptoms that predict microscopic pyuria. *Int Urogynecol J* 2018; 29(7): 1019-28.

13. Huang B, Zhang L, Zhang W, *et al*. Direct detection and identification of bacterial pathogens from urine with optimized specimen processing and enhanced testing algorithm. *J Clin Microbiol* 2017; 55(5): 1488-95.

14. Khasriya R, Khan S, Lunawat R, *et al*. The inadequacy of urinary dipstick and microscopy as surrogate markers of urinary tract infection in urological outpatients with lower urinary tract symptoms without acute frequency and dysuria. *J Urol* 2010; 183(5): 1843-7.

15. Kupelian AS, Horsley H, Khasriya R, *et al*. Discrediting microscopic pyuria and leucocyte esterase as diagnostic surrogates for infection in patients with lower urinary tract symptoms: results from a clinical and laboratory evaluation. *BJU Int* 2013; 112(2): 231-8.

16. Linder BJ, Bass EJ, Mostafid H, Boorjian SA. Guideline of guidelines: asymptomatic microscopic haematuria. *BJU Int* 2018; 121(2): 176-83.

17. Cumberbatch MGK, Jubber I, Black PC, *et al*. Epidemiology of bladder cancer: a systematic review and contemporary update of risk factors in 2018. *Eur Urol* 2018; 74(6): 784-95.

18. Schmitz-Drager BJ, Kuckuck EC, Zuiverloon TC, *et al*. Microhematuria assessment an IBCN consensus — based upon a critical review of current guidelines. *Urol Oncol* 2016; 34(10): 437-51.

19. Cara-Fuentes G, Clapp WL, Johnson RJ, Garin EH. Pathogenesis of proteinuria in idiopathic minimal change disease: molecular mechanisms. *Pediatr Nephrol* 2016; 31(12): 2179-89.

20. Berthet A, Bartolo S, Subtil D, *et al*. Spot urine protein-to-creatinine ratio as a diagnostic test in pre-eclampsia: a gold standard? *Int J Gynaecol Obstet* 2020; 149(1): 76-81.

21. Hamadah AM, Gharaibeh K, Mara KC, *et al*. Urinalysis for the diagnosis of glomerulonephritis: role of dysmorphic red blood cells. *Nephrol Dial Transplant* 2018; 33(8): 1397-403.

22. Browne RF, Zwirewich C, Torreggiani WC. Imaging of urinary tract infection in the adult. *Eur Radiol* 2004; 14 Suppl 3: E168-83.

23. Collins L, Sathiananthamoorthy S, Fader M, Malone-Lee J. Intermittent catheterisation after botulinum toxin injections: the time to reassess our practice. *Int Urogynecol J* 2017; 28(9): 1351-6.

24. Latthe P, Middleton L, Rachaneni S, *et al*. Ultrasound bladder wall thickness and detrusor overactivity: a multicentre test accuracy study. *BJOG* 2017; 124(9): 1422-9.

25. Liao L, Zhang F, Chen G. New grading system for upper urinary tract dilation using magnetic resonance urography in patients with neurogenic bladder. *BMC Urol* 2014; 14: 38.

26. van Nieuwkoop C, Hoppe BP, Bonten TN, *et al*. Predicting the need for radiologic imaging in adults with febrile urinary tract infection. *Clin Infect Dis* 2010; 51(11): 1266-72.

27. Brisbane W, Bailey MR, Sorensen MD. An overview of kidney stone imaging techniques. *Nat Rev Urol* 2016; 13(11) :654-62.

28. Paterson A. Urinary tract infection: an update on imaging strategies. *Eur Radiol* 2004; 14 Suppl 4: L89-100.

29. Frewen WK. An objective assessment of the unstable bladder of psychosomatic origin. *Br J Urol* 1978; 50(4): 246-9.

30. Byrne DJ, Stewart PA, Gray BK. The role of urodynamics in female urinary stress incontinence. *Br J Urol* 1987; 59(3): 228-9.

31. Buck AC, Castro JE, Chisholm GD. Proceedings: the value of urodynamics in the differential diagnosis of urinary outflow tract obstruction. *Br J Surg* 1974; 61(4): 329.

32. Schafer W, Abrams P, Liao L, *et al*. Good urodynamic practices: uroflowmetry, filling cystometry, and pressure-flow studies. *Neurourol Urodyn* 2002; 21(3): 261-74.

33. Blaivas JG. The bladder is an unreliable witness. *Neurourol Urodyn* 1996; 15(5): 443-5.

34. Malone-Lee JG, Al-Buheissi S. Does urodynamic verification of overactive bladder determine treatment success? Results from a randomized placebo-controlled study. *BJU Int* 2009; 103(7): 931-7.

35. Nager CW, Brubaker L, Litman HJ, *et al*. A randomized trial of urodynamic testing before stress-incontinence surgery. *N Engl J Med* 2012; 366(21): 1987-97.

36. Idriz S, Kirkham A, Rickards D, Malone-Lee JG. The failure of cystometric pressure/flow plots in characterising bladder outflow obstruction. *BJU Int* 2007; 99: 40-1.

37. Malde S, Palmisani S, Al-Kaisy A, Sahai A. Guideline of guidelines: bladder pain syndrome. *BJU Int* 2018; 122(5): 729-43.

38. West JB, Tsukimoto K, Mathieu-Costello O, Prediletto R. Stress failure in pulmonary capillaries. *J Appl Physiol* 1991; 70(4): 1731-42.

39. Wennevik GE, Meijlink JM, Hanno P, Nordling J. The role of glomerulations in bladder pain syndrome: a review. *J Urol* 2016; 195(1): 19-25.

40. Lynes WL, Flynn SD, Shortliffe LD, Stamey TA. The histology of interstitial cystitis. *Am J Surg Pathol* 1990; 14(10): 969-76.

41. Tomaszewski JE, Landis JR, Russack V, *et al*. Biopsy features are associated with primary symptoms in interstitial cystitis: results from the interstitial cystitis database study. *Urology* 2001; 57(6 Suppl 1): 67-81.

42. Dundore PA, Schwartz AM, Semerjian H. Mast cell counts are not useful in the diagnosis of nonulcerative interstitial cystitis. *J Urol* 1996; 155(3): 885-7.

43. Cornish J, Vanderwee MA, Ormrod DJ, Miller TE. Mucosal mast cells as a component of the inflammatory response to lower-urinary tract infection. *Int Arch Allergy Immunol* 1986; 81(4): 337-42.

44. Shaikh N, Borrell JL, Evron J, Leeflang MM. Procalcitonin, C-reactive protein, and erythrocyte sedimentation rate for the diagnosis of acute pyelonephritis in children. *Cochrane Database Syst Rev* 2015; 1: CD009185.

45. Ayazi P, Mahyar A, Daneshi MM, *et al*. Diagnostic accuracy of the quantitative C-reactive protein, erythrocyte sedimentation rate and white blood cell count in urinary tract infections among infants and children. *Malays J Med Sci* 2013; 20(5): 40-6.

Chapter 6

What cystitis does to you

In early 2019 the science correspondent of *The Guardian*, Hannah Devlin, brought our attention to anecdotal reports that implied the incidence of chronic cystitis was on the rise in the UK. Later that year she published an article on this (https://www.theguardian.com/society/2019/oct/04/rise-in-persistent-urinary-tract-infections-could-be-linked-to-antibiotics-crackdown). We had been aware of similar observations from clinical colleagues. Prompted by Hannah, with assistance from a data-savvy patient, we studied this.

NHS Digital (https://digital.nhs.uk) provides a rich source of aggregate data in the public domain obtained from provider and commissioner returns. We collected these data in order to examine the trends in the presentation of cystitis and IC/BPS/PBS over the 18 years of available data.

We obtained data for the years 1998 to 2016 for the diagnostic categories outlined in ▨ Table 6.1.

Table 6.1. The International Classification of Diseases (ICD) codes and diagnoses for which data were extracted from NHS Digital data stores.

N30.0	Acute cystitis
N30.1	Interstitial cystitis (chronic)
N30.2	Other chronic cystitis
N30.8	Other cystitis
N30.9	Cystitis, unspecified

We also obtained prescribing data from the primary care data available on the NHS site.

Figure 6.1 addresses hospital admissions but outpatient attendances are the same. We are experiencing a marked rise in the incidence of IC/BPS/PBS and it requires explanation.

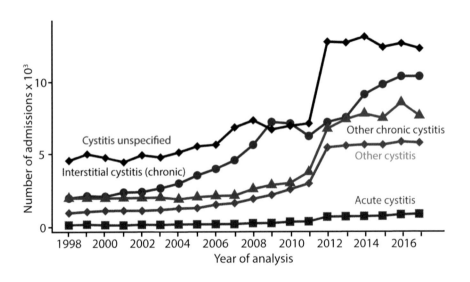

Figure 6.1. NHS admissions for cystitis diagnoses 1998 to 2016.

The diagnostic coding could be clearer but nevertheless the rise in the incidence of chronic and other recorded types of cystitis is well shown. This gains pace from 2002 which is when the first guidelines advocated 3-day antibiotic courses for acute cystitis followed by treatment based on culture. Whatever the explanation we have a growing problem since the millennium.

Figure 6.2 shows that the number of prescription scripts for nitrofurantoin increase but the number of tablets/capsules dispensed per script decreases; this translates as significantly more prescriptions but for shorter courses. Figure 6.3 provides a similar analysis for the use of trimethoprim which was used much more than nitrofurantoin in 1998.

Figure 6.1 implies that something has gone wrong. The rise in cases reflects a great amount of patient suffering, some of it life-changing. If your response is to blame AMR you are correct but perversely, in a manner that contradicts popular assumptions. We are going to explore the problem in this chapter through an analysis of the pathophysiology of UTI.

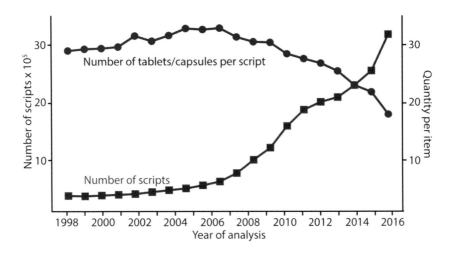

Figure 6.2. NHS data on nitrofurantoin prescriptions 1998 to 2016.

If we write a prescription for nitrofurantoin 100mg twice daily for 3 days it will be one item but the quantity will be 6, 100mg capsules. The same prescription for 14 days will be a quantity of 28, 100mg capsules. This graph shows that the quantity per item is falling from shorter duration of prescriptions but the number of prescriptions (items) is on the rise. The guidelines have influenced practice.

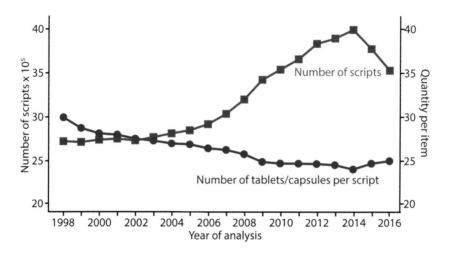

Figure 6.3. NHS data on trimethoprim prescriptions 1998 to 2016.

This figure shows a similar pattern to Figure 6.2 but from trimethoprim. There is a difference in that trimethoprim was much prescribed in 1998 which was not the case with nitrofurantoin. Recent years has seen a rise in the prescription items for trimethoprim but a fall in the quantity of tablets for each prescription.

A clue is found on the time axis of ▓ Figure 6.1. The European Association of Urology (EAU) guidelines on UTI [1] came out in 2001 and there followed a slew of others from competing organisations, which led to the enforcement of a 3-day treatment course for acute cystitis, with all subsequent treatment decisions based on the MSU culture data. The influence of the guidelines is demonstrated in ▓ Figures 6.2 and 6.3. This records a rise in quantity of the first-line UTI antibiotics nitrofurantoin and trimethoprim prescribed. Note how the ratio quantity: number of prescriptions betrays an intriguing trend. Whilst these antibiotics are being prescribed in shortened courses, the number of prescriptions has risen.

The advice on the treatment of acute UTI is based on RCTs of antibiotic treatment and their meta-analyses. The studies are reassuringly abundant, the majority funded by the pharmaceutical industry. Meta-analyses license the guideline panels to claim grade 1A evidence. But are the data of such quality? Whilst some meta-analyses boast success rates of 84% to 100% for 3-day and 14-day antibiotic treatments [2], buried in other data is evidence of microbiological and symptomatic failure in between 28% and 37% of patients within 4 to 14 weeks of treatment [3]. Many RCT publications report the positive findings, but the bad news is brushed away with Ockham's broom [4]. Do we tell our patients that our guideline treatment of UTI carries a 25% to 35% failure rate? Do we have contingencies for the unlucky? Can we find a warning in the guidelines?

Acute UTI is common and the cause of many antibiotic prescriptions (Figures 6.2 and 6.3). Thus, it attracts the attention of the campaigners combatting AMR. This is not a bad thing, but in dealing with the complexity of human disease it is important to adopt an approach more nuanced than a pickaxe. AMR initiatives tend to entail single-minded insistence on reducing antibiotic use for UTI. The principal tools are policing of guideline compliance and relying on urine culture as an arbiter between UTI and no UTI. In this world a negative culture is synonymous with no infection and an absolute contraindication to treatment of the symptoms with antibiotics. Regrettably, the urine culture is hopelessly insensitive and misses numerous, genuine UTIs [5, 6]; it is incapable of the task it has been delegated. Thus, we suspect that the widespread imposition of guidelines for the management of acute UTI has resulted in the increase in patients suffering from chronic UTI.

Figure 6.4 provides a plot of the admissions for the pooled diagnoses under the banner of chronic cystitis. We have marked in the publication dates of the various guidelines on cystitis which rain down like a ticker-tape parade. Every one of these persist with short courses of antibiotics for acute UTI, followed by management based on MSU culture. It's Nero-like, as all the while an alarming surge in these admissions gathers pace.

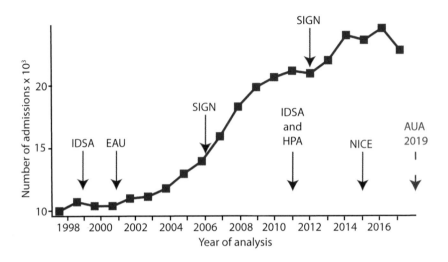

IDSA   Infectious Diseases Society of America

EAU   European Association of Urology

SIGN   Scottish Intercollegiate Guidelines Network

HPA   Health Protection Agency

NICE   National Institute for Health and Care Excellence

AUA   American Urological Association

Figure 6.4. NHS admissions for all cystitis diagnoses 1998 to 2017.

This figure has combined the admissions figures under a chronic cystitis umbrella and the notable rise in the incidence of these events is well shown. We have included the points where guidelines on cystitis have been published. They all perseverate, promoting short antibiotic courses for acute UTI with no consideration of the known failure rates. It seems that the advice for managing disappointing outcomes is to go by the cultures which have a high probability of being negative.

Most know the often stated claim that 80% of UTIs are caused by *E. coli* and that the causative microbes travel from the intestines via the perineum. These beliefs hinge on culture data, the belief that the normal bladder is sterile, and that microbes isolated are identified precisely at species level: none are true, so the surmised model does not seem convincing. *E. coli* is most easy to culture so is likely to be a frequent isolate.

Contradicting widely adopted practice should not be done lightly and we have a serious duty to justify our case soberly with solid empirical evidence. The MSU culture may be defective but that does not mean that patients with symptoms and signs and negative culture do not have UTI. Not presuming, we must scrutinise this with care.

All clinical science should start with the basic biology. With UTI our current knowledge depends much on experiments using *E. coli* conducted in mice [7]. We need to enhance these data by mounting complementary studies in humans. *E. coli* may not be the only offender [5, 8, 9] and a murine model reflects the human situation poorly [10].

We decided to use consilience to study this conundrum because it seemed to be so well suited to the clinical circumstance. Consilience [11], which we illustrate in ▨ Figure 6.5, is a powerful technique for getting to the truth. It is based on the principle that evidence from different independent sources will converge on a hypothesis if it is valid. If witnesses with disparate provenances agree then useful conclusions can be achieved. If you study ▨ Figure 6.5 you will see that we have covered a certain amount of the ground in the previous chapter. All of the time our focus has been on patients with chronic recalcitrant bladder pain and recurrent cystitis with negative routine urine culture. ▨ Figure 6.5 emphasises the fact that we have many more options than routine culture, cystoscopy and biopsy with which to make sense of this problem.

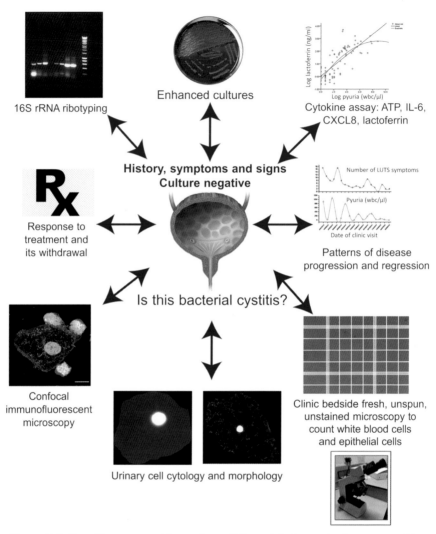

16S rRNA ribotyping

Enhanced cultures

Cytokine assay: ATP, IL-6, CXCL8, lactoferrin

History, symptoms and signs
Culture negative

Response to treatment and its withdrawal

Patterns of disease progression and regression

Is this bacterial cystitis?

Confocal immunofluorescent microscopy

Clinic bedside fresh, unspun, unstained microscopy to count white blood cells and epithelial cells

Urinary cell cytology and morphology

Figure 6.5. Consilience — evidence from different independent sources will converge on a valid hypothesis. If evidence from disparate provenances agree, it is strong validation.

Consilience is a powerful technique when you do not have the access that is allowed through animal studies. We surround our problem with "eyes" that scrutinise the matter from different, independent perspectives. The more that the observations prove commensurate the greater the probability that our conclusions approach the truth. The disparate perspectives may also alert us to a problem with your current beliefs because of a discordant result.

126

The pathophysiology of UTI

An acute urine infection causes distressing symptoms and signs so the causative pathogens must be invading the tissues of the bladder and not just swimming around in the urine. The urothelium is in the line of attack and we should look to that to study the events. Thus, in █ Figure 6.6, we provide some graphical images to aid the ensuing description. The various stages outlined in █ Figure 6.6 are initiated by an acute infection. The overwhelming majority of people get over these without difficulty. This means that the model that we describe must be prone to abort but whilst there are some hints coming through, we do not yet understand the mechanism of that occurrence or what causes the infection to develop into a chronic parasitisation.

E. coli, which are the most studied bacteria of UTI, bear tentacles called pili or fimbriae (singular pilus/fimbria). A subset is termed "Type 1 pili". These carry sticky, adhesin molecules (aka adhesion molecules) called FimH. These bind with a mannose-containing glycoprotein receptor [12] on the surface of the urothelial cells lining the urinary tract.

Stage 1

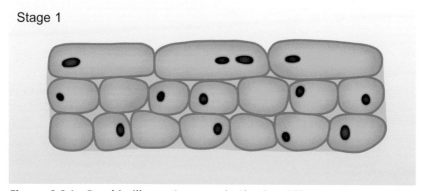

Figure 6.6.1. Graphic illustrations to clarify the different elements that make up a UTI. Whilst these are demonstrated as different stages, they may occur at similar times in different parts of the urothelium. The superficial umbrella cell layer is at the top where it is seen that this can be multinucleated. Because the sections show a 2D version of a 3D anatomy the nuclei do not always show. *Illustration courtesy of Alex Wilby.*

Stage 2

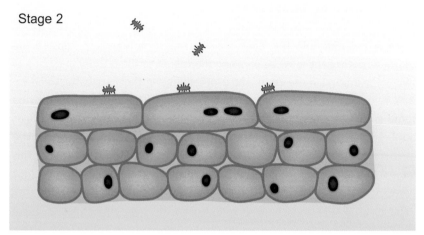

Figure 6.6.2. We have bacteria with their fimbriae approaching the urothelial cells and binding to the surfaces. In the case of *E. coli*, Type 1 pili will bind to a mannose-containing glycoprotein receptor. Whether urinary mannose can block this or not is uncertain and other microbes may bind to other receptors. *Illustration courtesy of Alex Wilby.*

Stage 3

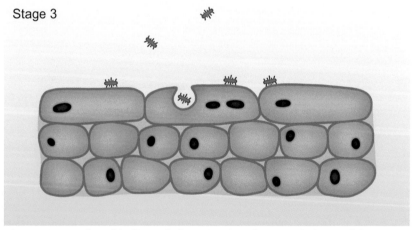

Figure 6.6.3. After binding of the microbe the cytoskeleton deforms to enable the microbe to be engulfed by the cell in much the same way that a macrophage works. It may be a defence mechanism but the microbes have evolved to subvert it to their advantage. *Illustration courtesy of Alex Wilby.*

Stage 4

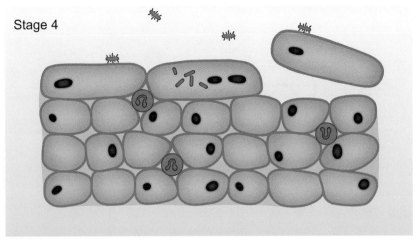

Figure 6.6.4. The microbes inside the cell have shed their fimbriae and have started to divide in some cases. An innate immune reaction ensues with the arrival of white blood cells. The urothelium starts to thicken with the laying down of more cells and the exfoliation of cells starts to develop particularly with the shedding of parasitised cells. It is a way of getting rid of the infection. *Illustration courtesy of Alex Wilby.*

Stage 5

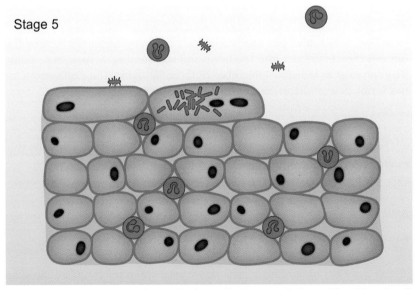

Figure 6.6.5. The urothelium thickens further and the white blood cell infiltration increases with overflow into the urine. The exfoliation of the cells results in ulceration. *Illustration courtesy of Alex Wilby.*

Stage 6

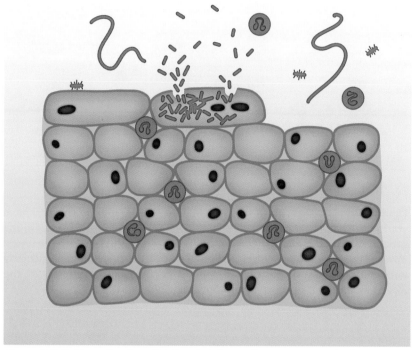

Figure 6.6.6. The microbes dividing inside a cell may eventually destroy the cell and then break out into the urine and surrounding tissues. In so doing they can exist as individual microbes or form filaments. The explanation for this is not clear. *Illustration courtesy of Alex Wilby.*

The binding stimulates the cytoskeleton, the structural scaffold of the cell, to envelope the bacterium and draw it inside where, strictly speaking, it is supposed to be butchered. However, pathogens have evolved to survive, hijack the cell, and use the cell's content to reproduce. In this circumstance the bacteria will divide, fill the cell, destroy it, breaking out into the tissues and urine and then search out fresh, new cells to infect similarly.

The parasitising bacteria may do something else: they are able to manipulate the cell to create an abode in which they can survive in a dormant state. Additionally, some microbes may use quorum sensing to communicate,

Stage 7

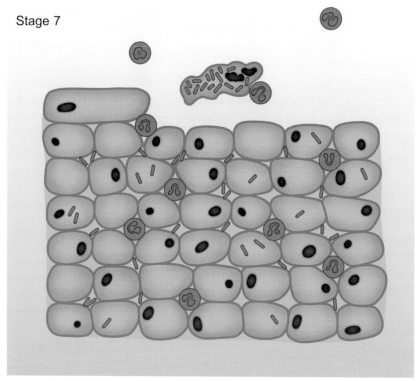

Figure 6.6.7. The infection may spread through the inter-cell spaces travelling down to infect cells at all levels. Much of the parasitisation will result in quiescent microbes shielding themselves in biofilms inside the cells and remaining dormant without dividing. The urothelium continues to thicken and cells whether healthy, parasitised or dying are shed into the urine. *Illustration courtesy of Alex Wilby.*

thereby building a band of compatriots embedded in a protective mucous barrier, thus forming a biofilm which may exist inside or on the cell surface [13]. All normal biological surfaces support biofilms; this is a natural process, not intrinsically pathological. For example, normal oral and vaginal biofilms may protect against Candida infection [14].

The resting pathogens are protected from immune and antibiotic attack by their host cells, the impenetrable properties of the biofilms and by not dividing, since antibiotics act on dividing bacteria [15]. These microbes are aptly called "persisters" and are antibiotic-resistant infections waiting to break out and cause an acute infection, aka an acute flare [16, 17]. It may be that persisters are the cause of chronic recalcitrant bladder pain and recurrent cystitis; it is an occurrence that we should seek to prevent [18-20].

Murine studies have found that, during the first exposure to infection, the pathogens may alter the urothelial cell functions so as to increase susceptibility to future infection and creation of persister colonies [21, 22]. In mice at least, the initial infection must span between 2 and 14 days before this mechanism becomes active [23]. The process can be aborted by prompt

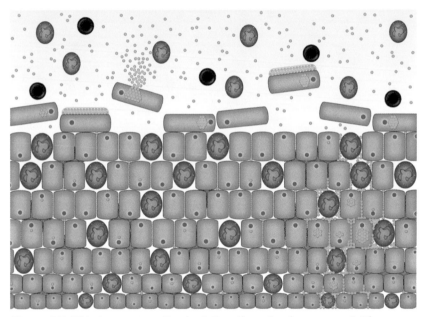

Figure 6.7. This is a composite depicting the microbes as cocci. There are dilated blood vessels which will inflame the urothelium. They are friable and will break if stretched. The urothelium is much thickened with white blood cell infiltrates. There are white blood cells, red blood cells and bacteria in the urine. Cells are shedding from the surface but clumps may come away leaving deep ulceration. Note the widespread parasitisation, including surface formation of biofilms. To the right there are intracellular microbes waking up, dividing and gradually overwhelming their host cell which they then abandon to divide through the interspaces seeking new homes. *Illustration courtesy of Alex Wilby.*

treatment in the first 24 hours. The duration of this window of opportunity, beyond 24 hours, is not yet known. Once the biofilms and intracellular persisters are established it is difficult to clear them.

Figure 6.7 provides a composite of the various active elements in these infections. These illustrations can be helpful in understanding a complex situation but beware of their ability to oversimplify the story and encourage a naïve perception of what is afoot. We have therefore provided some additional images that bring the reality to the fore.

Figures 6.8 to 6.11 are confocal micrographs obtained in our laboratories from patients who had been diagnosed with IC/PBS/BPS. These capture that behaviour of white blood cells, bacteria and epithelial cells. In subsequent chapters we shall describe the differences in measures of these cells that contrast with normal controls.

Figures 6.8 and 6.9 show an image of two infected urothelial cells. We know it to be infected because two neutrophils appear to be attacking the cell-associated microbes and three others are approaching the scene. An important mechanism is caught where a microbe is seen to be exiting the cell whilst stealing cell membrane with which to coat and protect itself. On the left of the figure are microbes that are not coated in cell membrane. There is another element to this image; at the overlap between the two cells there is some clustering of microbes. When this is examined in 3-D, it can be seen that these bacteria are tracking between the cells despite the existence of the tight junctions that bind the cells together. The microbes are much more numerous outside of the cells than inside.

Figure 6.10 illustrates a remarkable phenomenon — NETosis; the white blood cell expels its DNA and thereby forms a fishing net that traps bacteria which are then destroyed by enzymatic action.

Figure 6.11 shows two white blood cells that are attacking microbes in the urine. The white blood cell to the left has declumped its DNA in preparation to extruding it into a net in the process of NETosis.

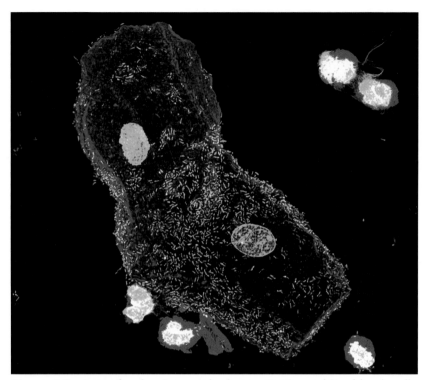

Figure 6.8. A confocal micrograph demonstrating white blood cells attacking parasitising microbes with some bacteria escaping and coating themselves in protective cell membrane. DAPI staining of the DNA makes the nuclei and bacteria turn green. The cell membrane is stained pink by wheat germ agglutinin. At 9 o'clock at the outer margin of the cell there is a microbe coated in membrane. The white blood cells are attacking parasitising microbes, with some bacteria escaping and coating themselves in protective cell membrane. There is clustering of bacteria at the join between the cells. 3D imaging shows these to be crowding the intercellular space where they have disrupted the tight junctions. *Micrograph courtesy of Harry Horsley.*

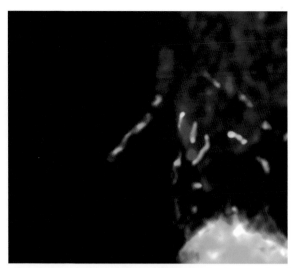

Figure 6.9. This close-up of a confocal micrograph shows microbes escaping the urothelial cell; in the process they are stealing pink-stained cell membrane which they use to protect themselves. The host membrane coating may protect them from immune attack because they may be mistaken for host tissue. *Micrograph courtesy of Harry Horsley.*

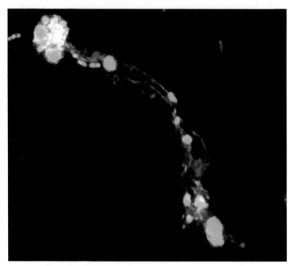

Figure 6.10. A confocal micrograph demonstrating a white blood cell which has expelled its DNA and thereby fashioned a net which is trapping microbes in its mesh. These will be destroyed. It is similar to the way that spiders use their webs. *Micrograph courtesy of Harry Horsley.*

135

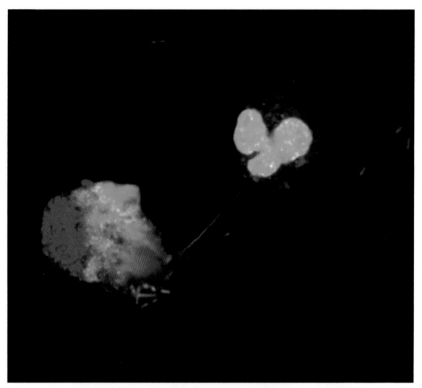

Figure 6.11. A confocal micrograph demonstrating two white blood cells that are attacking microbes in the urine. The white blood cell to the left has declumped its DNA in preparation to extruding it into a net in the process of NETosis. *Micrograph courtesy of Harry Horsley.*

These confocal micrographs, obtained from patients with cUTI symptoms and signs, but with negative cultures and therefore diagnosed with IC, capture important pathological occurrences that show attacks on uroepithelial cells by microbes, their parasitisation and the counter-measures taken by the immune-mediated white blood cells. The bacteria are caught *in flagrante* attacking the host cells. It is not tenable to waive it all away with *ad hoc* contrivances invoking autoimmunity, allergy or mast cell activation which are all used to account for IC/PBS/BPS without pathophysiological evidence.

The histopathology of cystitis can be difficult to follow for us who are not histopathologists, so to help us all we have prepared some images that abstract the salient features from micrographs. The original micrographs that modelled for these pictures are to be found on the American Urological Association's excellent pathology site at: https://www.auanet.org/education/auauniversity/education-products-and-resources/pathology-for-urologists/urinary-bladder/cystitis/follicular-cystitis. It is well worth a visit.

▓ Figure 6.12 illustrates a normal bladder with the three layers of the epithelial cells. Note that the submucosa contains, amongst other elements, blood capillaries, fibroblasts, leucocytes, macrophages, lymphocytes and

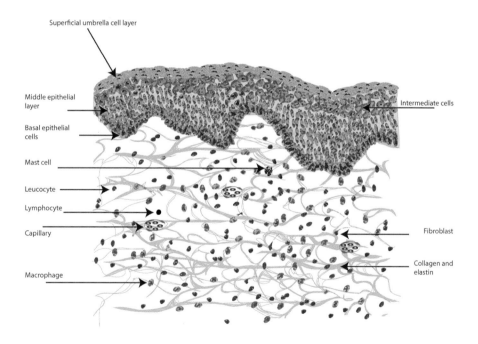

Figure 6.12. The histology of the normal bladder. Note the depth of the epithelial cell layer with the stacked palisade of cells moving up from the basal layer. There are immune cells, including mast cells, patrolling the submucosa. *Illustration by James Malone-Lee.*

mast cells. The mast cells are supposed to be there. Note how the epithelium is multi-layered and the cells change into the flattened superficial umbrella cells. The capillaries are not stuffed with red cells.

Figure 6.13 shows the initial response to an infection causing a chronic inflammatory response. There is metaplasia of the epithelium and exfoliation of cells. The urothelial thickening would account for the ultrasound

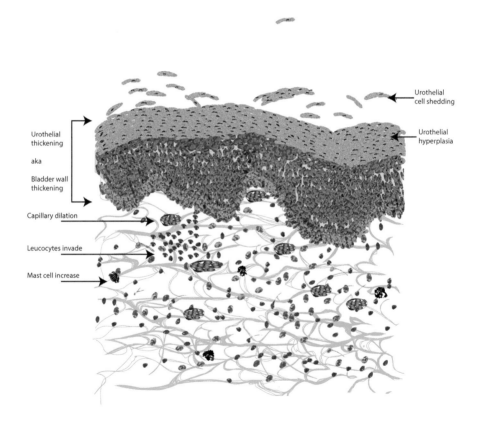

Figure 6.13. An early response to parasitisation of the uroepithelial cells by bacteria is metaplastic change with thickening of the urothelium, exfoliation of cells with shedding into the urine and increased cell turnover. The capillaries dilate and being friable will bleed easily. There is an infiltration of white blood cells; later lymphocytes and mast cells will also be present. *Illustration by James Malone-Lee.*

appearance of bladder wall thickening. The capillaries are filled with blood cells and clusters of white blood cells have arrived. Note that there are scattered mast cells similarly to other acute inflammatory reactions in other tissues. There are no clusters of mast cells which feature in the mast cell disorders.

We have provided ▦ Figure 6.14 in order to explain the significance of von Brunn's nests, cystitis cystica, nodular cystitis and eosinophilic cystitis. The first two are seen in normal circumstances as well as in association with cystitis. They are non-specific changes that are not indicative of particular

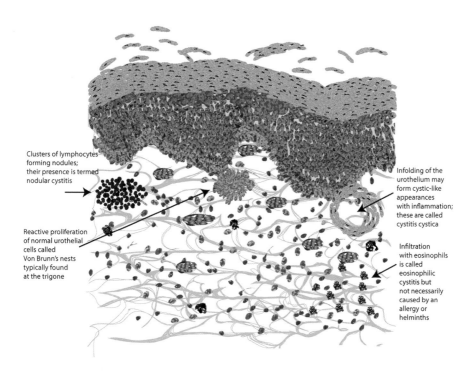

Clusters of lymphocytes forming nodules; their presence is termed nodular cystitis

Reactive proliferation of normal urothelial cells called Von Brunn's nests typically found at the trigone

Infolding of the urothelium may form cystic-like appearances with inflammation; these are called cystitis cystica

Infiltration with eosinophils is called eosinophilic cystitis but not necessarily caused by an allergy or helminths

Figure 6.14. There are some histological appearances that may be referred to in a bladder wall biopsy report: "cystitis cystica", "von Brunn's nests", "nodular cystitis" and "eosinophilic cystitis". These are not specific forms of cystitis; they are just variations in the form of the inflammatory response. *Illustration by James Malone-Lee.*

diseases. Patients may be diagnosed with cystitis cystica but that is not to imply a separate clinical entity.

⬜ Figure 6.15 charts the progression of the cystitis with the greater infiltration of white blood cells/leucocytes forming microabscesses which may be painful. Whilst these changes are developing it should not be forgotten that the microbes will be parasitising the urothelial cells as illustrated in the ⬜ Figure 6.6 series above.

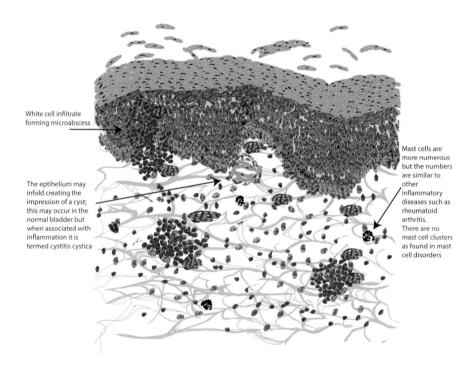

White cell infiltrate forming microabscess

The eptihelium may infold creating the impression of a cyst; this may occur in the normal bladder but when associated with inflammation it is termed cystitis cystica

Mast cells are more numerous but the numbers are similar to other inflammatory diseases such as rheumatoid arthritis. There are no mast cell clusters as found in mast cell disorders

Figure 6.15. As the inflammatory reaction progresses the exfoliation of the urothelial cells and urothelial thickening increases. Microabscesses form and these will be painful as with any pustule. The patient may feel particularly unwell with systemic symptoms. The distribution of mast cells is not different from many other chronic inflammatory states. *Illustration by James Malone-Lee.*

▓ Figure 6.16 shows the occurrence of epithelial ulceration with bleeding from the exposed submucosa. If you stretch the bladder when the capillaries are so filled they are going to rupture and bleed which is a reasonable

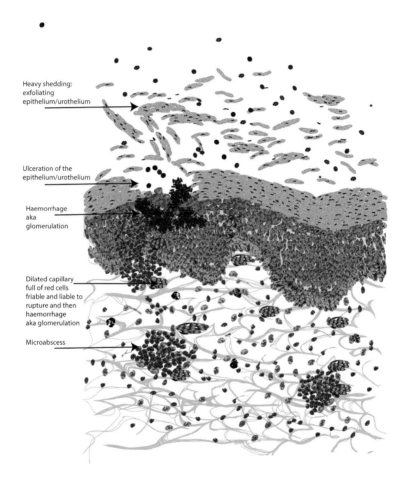

Figure 6.16. As the infection and inflammation continue unabated we see enlargement of the abscesses, ulceration of the uroepithelium and haemorrhage. Glomerulations are such haemorrhages. These changes are little different from a Hunner's ulcer, so there is a pressing need for work that seeks out clearer differentiation between the two states. *Illustration by James Malone-Lee.*

explanation for glomerulations. The histology of Hunner's ulcers features all of these elements, so further efforts at differentiation from other acute and chronic inflammation is overdue. The pathology sabotages the plausibility of instillations of GAG layer replacements. The uroepithelium is exfoliating, ulcerating and being washed with urine. What happens to a finger plaster when you go swimming? It rarely stays in place.

Bacteria, perturbing urothelial cells, trigger an innate immune response. This manifests all the features of acute and then chronic inflammation [23]. There is pyuria, an inflammatory infiltrate of the urothelium and cytokine activation.

The urothelium carries receptors able to recognise malevolent microbes by binding to "pathogen-associated molecular patterns" (PAMPs); the Toll-like receptor (TLR) family is the most studied, particularly bacterial adherence to TLR4 receptors. *In vivo* studies of bacterial invasion of urothelial cells chart a rapid cytokine response involving several cytokines, notably the acute inflammatory reactants, ATP, IL-6, IL-8 (CXCL8) and lactoferrin.

ATP is an important urothelial cell distress signal [24], and it is released by inflammatory cells [25] and bacteria. Increased ATP has also been shown to be released from cultured urothelial cells infected with uropathogenic *E. coli* (UPEC) [26, 27], and UPEC also produce ATP when cultured *in vitro* [28]. ATP is known to promote cell apoptosis, which has significance here. ATP levels reflect microbial biomass and in the food, water and sanitation industry, ATP levels are used as a measure of bacterial contamination [29]. As an aside, in fact water concentrations of *E. coli* are used to measure human faecal contamination. The commonest cause of travellers' diarrhoea is *E. coli* infection, so if you have experienced this it was because you inadvertently drank a suspension of someone else's faeces. That should make you feel champion.

IL-6 has numerous actions but it is a pro-inflammatory cytokine promoting the acute phase, the innate immune response. IL-6 is detected in the urine in most patients with positive urine cultures but it was only detected in the serum of symptomatic patients [30], so it would seem that there are local and systemic cytokine roles. Studies have shown that IL-6 production increases neutrophil migration and activation of IL-8 (CXCL8) [31, 32].

IL-8 (CXCL8) causes neutrophils to migrate towards the infection location and it stimulates them to act as phagocytes that engulf the bacteria.

Lactoferrin sequesters free iron, depriving bacteria of an essential nutrient [33]. It has other antimicrobial properties: it binds to lipopolysaccharide (LPS) of the bacterial wall catalysing membrane oxidation and bacterial lysis [33]. It stimulates phagocytes and interferes with proton translocation through the cell membrane disrupting microbial attachment capacity [34, 35]. It is thought that the dominant mechanism of action is via its iron binding properties and interaction with LPS of the bacterial cell wall [36]; bacteria need iron to thrive.

Gram-negative bacteria binding to TLR4 receptors stimulate mast cells to release a number of pro-inflammatory cytokines, including TNFα, IL-1 and IL-6 without degranulation. Gram-positive bacteria promote degranulation and histamine release; these increase vascular permeability and recruit immunocytes to fight infection [37]. If mast cells degranulate under the epithelium they stimulate exfoliation of infected urothelial cells [38]. There is no need to invent a mast cell activation disorder or other pathology to explain their involvement; they fight infection, so subverting this with antihistamines and similar agents does not make sense.

It is well recognised that urothelium perturbed by infection will increase turnover and exfoliate large numbers of cells [23, 39-42]. This is a good option if parasitisation of these cells is active. It would seem to be the principal method for clearing the urinary tract of the parasitised urothelial cells. We have shown this phenomenon consistently in association with UTI and we monitor our patients' response to treatment by plotting the urinary white blood cell and epithelial cell counts. We were interested to discover that increased exfoliation of uroepithelial cells is a feature of normal human pregnancy [43]. Perhaps this is an evolved mechanism, deployed to protect against UTI. After all, urinary tract infection in pregnancy is associated with miscarriage, preterm birth, small babies and pyelonephritis. The fact that mast cells play a part in this exfoliative response to infection makes us wonder whether the preoccupation with mast cells in interstitial cystitis might be a blind alley.

We have examined the cytokines, lactoferrin, IL-6, CXCL8 and ATP and found them to be associated with pyuria and increased bacterial culture isolates [44]. These are correlations of pathophysiological interest; we have never advocated the measurements for a clinical diagnostic role but they have played a powerful role in discrediting dipsticks and MSU culture, demonstrating mischief afoot when the latter tests tried to reassure.

The syndrome of chronic UTI

So what do we think is going on? We may only answer that by cautiously explaining what appears most probable, given current evidence, from animal and human studies. It is an important distinction. These beliefs are temporary, contingent and certain to be modified, given new evidence.

The model that we follow at this time is as follows: acute urinary tract infection may well be cleared by the innate immune response but this is not guaranteed and in that situation an antibiotic prescription is necessary. Whether that be taken for 3 days or 14 days, the RCTs of antibiotic treatment of UTI show that there is a 25% to 35% risk of such treatment failing. There is evidence that failure to treat a UTI promptly opens the door to successful, long-term parasitisation of urothelial cells. This can involve microbes embedded in surface biofilms or intracellular colonies similarly protected by a biofilm matrix. In parasitising a cell, the microbes may co-opt the cell's chemistry to serve their reproduction and in so doing destroy their host. There is another pathway that causes the microbe to enter a dormant state and not divide but to use the host cell to protect and sustain it. These microbes are called persisters and they are protected by the cell. They are impervious to antibiotic attack by reason of their biofilm and not dividing. Such persister microbes have methods for moving to fresh cells when necessary, so that they can achieve a chronic, antibiotic-resistant infection lasting for years.

We do not know why some people shake off an acute urine infection using their innate immunity alone. Apart from antimicrobial resistance, why do some respond to treatment with antibiotics and others do not? Why do some develop chronic urothelial colonisation whereas others escape this? What steps can we take to prevent chronic infection? We do not have the answers to these pressing questions.

In our laboratory we have noticed that perturbation of a parasitised cell, be it physical or chemical, may stimulate a sleeping microbe to bestir and start dividing with its progeny packing the cell which is destroyed. A dividing microbial swarm is released, possibly causing an acute cystitis episode. This may be why sex, vaginal instrumentation, strenuous exercise, alcohol and specific foodstuffs cause acute flares of infection exacerbations in some patients, but we do not know that.

The microbes, whilst dormant, can still aggravate their host cell which remains capable of signalling its distress. Thus, a chronic inflammatory response may be mounted, challenging the chronic parasitisation. Because of the biofilms and the protection afforded by the host cell, this counter-attack may be insufficient to clear the infection but enough to cause the distressing symptoms associated with chronic cystitis. The urothelial cell exfoliation seems to be the only way of clearing the infection. Unfortunately, the offending microbes seem to have evolved means of subverting the immune mechanisms, although we have yet to discover that whole story. For example, Figure 6.9 captures some microbes dressing up as urothelial cells; that might be a means of camouflage to subvert immune recognition.

From a clinical perspective we have the makings for a nasty problem. Given an acute UTI, a clock starts and it seems that there is a time window during which this should be cleared or the chances of an intracellular parasitisation and chronic disease rise. Whilst our protocols encourage us to respond conservatively, they fail to alert us to a risk of potentially serious disease. If antibiotics are used it is short courses that are approved. It is not stated that the treatment failure rate is 25% and 35% and by the time this is realised sufficient time has elapsed to make a chronic infection more likely. Regrettably, the assessment of patients failing first-line treatment hinges on a urinalysis using dipsticks and/or urine culture. These two tests are discredited and proven to be insensitive and misleading. A consequence of their use is that a small minority of patients are exposed to risk of a chronic infection that is exceedingly difficult to erase, and can be life-changing. They will defy diagnosis because the tests that assess them are incompetent and imply that there is no infection present. On the contrary, we have shown that these patients demonstrate a host of inflammatory markers in the urine, pyuria, evidence of reactive urothelial metaplasia and parasitisation, and perturbation of the microbiome. Because the cultures are so commonly negative, they are diagnosed with interstitial cystitis, psychosomatic disease and other dubious constructs. All the while, this is a chronic disease so the numbers affected will continue to rise as new victims join the field.

Our suspicions are that the contemporary situation is the consequence of the blind adherence to dubious guidelines, the insistence on using discredited tests and antibiotic treatments curtailed by misplaced fear of AMR. This is an iatrogenic tragedy for the lives of so many victims.

What this means to the patient

To recap on some of this, at this time the most probable explanatory model is that patients experience an infection of the bladder that involves parasitisation of the lining urothelial cells going deep into the base of the urothelium. The affected cells signal their distress and an inflammatory reaction starts. The inflammation irritates the bladder causing frequency and urgency. Pain will also feature and the longer that the inflammation persists the more complex that experience. Pain can radiate to different parts of the pelvis, the vagina, legs and loins. Usually, patients describe relentless low-level symptoms punctuated by acute flares and that can be distressing. These outbreaks are interpreted as isolated acute urine infections, but the evidence points to exacerbations of the same chronic disease. A recurring feature of the history is that the patients, convinced of a urine infection, are confounded when their urine tests negative. The evidence implies that the patients' symptoms are accurate in indicating infection. This is a matter of much concern; we have to consider the probability that what the patients describe may be a most valid representation of their plight and we should recognise that.

References

1. Naber KG, Bergman B, Bishop MC, *et al*. EAU guidelines for the management of urinary and male genital tract infections. Urinary Tract Infection (UTI) Working Group of the Health Care Office (HCO) of the European Association of Urology (EAU). *Eur Urol* 2001; 40(5): 576-88.

2. Gupta K, Hooton TM, Naber KG, *et al*. International clinical practice guidelines for the treatment of acute uncomplicated cystitis and pyelonephritis in women: a 2010 update by the Infectious Diseases Society of America and the European Society for Microbiology and Infectious Diseases. *Clin Infect Dis* 2011; 52(5): e103-20.

3. Milo G, Katchman EA, Paul M, *et al*. Duration of antibacterial treatment for uncomplicated urinary tract infection in women. *Cochrane Database Syst Rev* 2005; 2: CD004682.

4. Dennett DC. *Intuition pumps and other tools for thinking*, 1st ed. New York: W. W. Norton & Company; 2013: 1-40.

5. Sathiananthamoorthy S, Malone-Lee J, Gill K, *et al*. Reassessment of routine midstream culture in diagnosis of urinary tract infection. *J Clin Microbiol* 2019; 57(3): 01452-18.

6. Gill K, Kang R, Sathiananthamoorthy S, *et al*. A blinded observational cohort study of the microbiological ecology associated with pyuria and overactive bladder symptoms. *Int Urogynecol J* 2018; 29(10): 1493-500.

7. Tenke P, Köves B, Nagy K, *et al*. Update on biofilm infections in the urinary tract. *World J Urol* 2012; 30(1): 51-7.

8. Thomas-White K, Forster SC, Kumar N, *et al*. Culturing of female bladder bacteria reveals an interconnected urogenital microbiota. *Nat Commun* 2018; 9(1): 1557.

9. Price TK, Hilt EE, Dune TJ, *et al*. Urine trouble: should we think differently about UTI? *Int Urogynecol J* 2018; 29(2): 205-10.

10. Parsons BA, Drake MJ. Animal models in overactive bladder research. *Handb Exp Pharmacol* 2011; 202: 15-43.

11. Wilson EO. *Consilience: the unity of knowledge*. London: Abacus; 1999.

12. Mulvey MA, Schilling JD, Hultgren SJ. Establishment of a persistent *Escherichia coli* reservoir during the acute phase of a bladder infection. *Infect Immun* 2001; 69(7): 4572-9.

13. Donlan RM. Biofilms: microbial life on surfaces. *Emerg Infect Dis* 2002; 8(9): 881-90.

14. McLean RJ. Normal bacterial flora may inhibit *Candida albicans* biofilm formation by Autoinducer-2. *Front Cell Infect Microbiol* 2014; 4: 117.

15. Blango MG, Mulvey MA. Persistence of uropathogenic *Escherichia coli* in the face of multiple antibiotics. *Antimicrob Agents Chemother* 2010; 54(5): 1855-63.

16. Lewis K. Persister cells. *Annu Rev Microbiol* 2010; 64: 357-72.

17. Maisonneuve E, Gerdes K. Molecular mechanisms underlying bacterial persisters. *Cell* 2014; 157(3): 539-48.

18. Anderson GG, Dodson KW, Hooton TM, Hultgren SJ. Intracellular bacterial communities of uropathogenic *Escherichia coli* in urinary tract pathogenesis. *Trends Microbiol* 2004; 12(9): 424-30.

19. Khasriya R, Sathiananthamoorthy S, Ismail S, *et al*. Spectrum of bacterial colonization associated with urothelial cells from patients with chronic lower urinary tract symptoms. *J Clin Microbiol* 2013; 51(7): 2054-62.

20. Horsley H, Malone-Lee J, Holland D, *et al*. *Enterococcus faecalis* subverts and invades the host urothelium in patients with chronic urinary tract infection. *PloS One* 2013; 8(12): e83637.

21. O'Brien VP, Hannan TJ, Yu L, *et al*. A mucosal imprint left by prior *Escherichia coli* bladder infection sensitizes to recurrent disease. *Nat Microbiol* 2016; 2: 16196.

22. O'Brien VP, Hannan TJ, Schaeffer AJ, Hultgren SJ. Are you experienced? Understanding bladder innate immunity in the context of recurrent urinary tract infection. *Curr Opin Infect Dis* 2015; 28(1): 97-105.

23. Hannan TJ, Mysorekar IU, Hung CS, *et al*. Early severe inflammatory responses to uropathogenic *E. coli* predispose to chronic and recurrent urinary tract infection. *PLoS Pathog* 2010; 6(8): e1001042.

24. Van der Wijk T, De Jonge HR, Tilly BC. Osmotic cell swelling-induced ATP release mediates the activation of extracellular signal-regulated protein kinase (Erk)-1/2 but not the activation of osmo-sensitive anion channels. *Biochem J* 1999; 343 Pt 3: 579-86.

25. van der Weyden L, Conigrave AD, Morris MB. Signal transduction and white cell maturation via extracellular ATP and the P2Y11 receptor. *Immunol Cell Biol* 2000; 78(4): 369-74.

26. Crane JK, Naeher TM, Choudhari SS, Giroux EM. Two pathways for ATP release from host cells in enteropathogenic *Escherichia coli* infection. *Am J Physiol Gastrointest Liver Physiol* 2005; 289(3): G407-17.

27. Save S, Persson K. Extracellular ATP and P2Y receptor activation induce a proinflammatory host response in the human urinary tract. *Infect Immun* 2010; 78(8): 3609-15.

28. Hanberger H, Nilsson LE, Kihlstrom E, Maller R. Postantibiotic effect of beta-lactam antibiotics on *Escherichia coli* evaluated by bioluminescence assay of bacterial ATP. *Antimicrob Agents Chemother* 1990; 34(1): 102-6.

29. Poulis JA, de Pijper M, Mossel DA, Dekkers PP. Assessment of cleaning and disinfection in the food industry with the rapid ATP-bioluminescence technique combined with the tissue

fluid contamination test and a conventional microbiological method. *Int J Food Microbiol* 1993; 20(2): 109-16.

30. Hedges S, Anderson P, Lidin-Janson G, *et al*. Interleukin-6 response to deliberate colonization of the human urinary tract with Gram-negative bacteria. *Infect Immun* 1991; 59(1): 421-7.

31. Sadik CD, Kim ND, Luster AD. Neutrophils cascading their way to inflammation. *Trends Immunol* 2011; 32(10): 452-60.

32. Mihara M, Hashizume M, Yoshida H, *et al*. IL-6/IL-6 receptor system and its role in physiological and pathological conditions. *Clin Sci (Lond)* 2012; 122(4): 143-59.

33. Farnaud S, Evans RW. Lactoferrin — a multifunctional protein with antimicrobial properties. *Mol Immunol* 2003; 40(7): 395-405.

34. Andrés MT, Fierro JF. Antimicrobial mechanism of action of transferrins: selective inhibition of H+-ATPase. *Antimicrob Agents Chemother* 2010; 54(10): 4335-42.

35. Bortner CA, Arnold RR, Miller RD. Bactericidal effect of lactoferrin on *Legionella pneumophila*: effect of the physiological state of the organism. *Can J Microbiol* 1989; 35(11): 1048-51.

36. Odell EW, Sarra R, Foxworthy M, *et al*. Antibacterial activity of peptides homologous to a loop region in human lactoferrin. *FEBS Lett* 1996; 382(1-2): 175-8.

37. Conti P, Carinci F, Caraffa A, *et al*. Link between mast cells and bacteria: antimicrobial defense, function and regulation by cytokines. *Med Hypotheses* 2017; 106: 10-4.

38. Choi HW, Bowen SE, Miao Y, *et al*. Loss of bladder epithelium induced by cytolytic mast cell granules. *Immunity* 2016; 45(6): 1258-69.

39. Dalal E, Medalia O, Harari O, Aronson M. Moderate stress protects female mice against bacterial infection of the bladder by eliciting uroepithelial shedding. *Infect Immun* 1994; 62(12): 5505-10.

40. Smith YC, Rasmussen SB, Grande KK, *et al*. Hemolysin of uropathogenic *Escherichia coli* evokes extensive shedding of the uroepithelium and hemorrhage in bladder tissue within the first 24 hours after intraurethral inoculation of mice. *Infect Immun* 2008; 76(7): 2978-90.

41. Thumbikat P, Berry RE, Zhou G, *et al*. Bacteria-induced uroplakin signaling mediates bladder response to infection. *PLoS Pathog* 2009; 5(5): e1000415.

42. Uchida K, Samma S, Rinsho K, *et al*. Stimulation of epithelial hyperplasia in rat urinary bladder by *Escherichia coli* cystitis. *J Urol* 1989; 142(4): 1122-6.

43. Liou N, Currie J, James C, *et al*. Urothelial cells may indicate underlying bacteriuria in pregnancy at term: a comparative study. *BMC Pregnancy Childbirth* 2017; 17(1): 414.

44.   Gill K, Horsley H, Kupelian AS, *et al*. Urinary ATP as an indicator of infection and inflammation of the urinary tract in patients with lower urinary tract symptoms. *BMC Urol* 2015; 15: 7.

Chapter 7

Treating the patient

Andrew Grove was born as András István Gróf, a Hungarian Jew. He summarised the first twenty years of his extraordinary life in his autobiography as follows:

"By the time I was twenty, I had lived through a Hungarian Fascist dictatorship, German military occupation, the Nazis' 'Final Solution', the siege of Budapest by the Soviet Red Army, a period of chaotic democracy in the years immediately after the war, a variety of repressive Communist regimes, and a popular uprising that was put down at gunpoint. Many young people were killed; countless others were interned. Some two hundred thousand Hungarians escaped to the West. I was one of them."

He arrived in New York in 1957 able to speak little English but in 1960 he was awarded a BSc in Chemical Engineering from City College of New York and a PhD from the University of California, Berkeley, in 1963. In 1967 he published a textbook, *Physics and Technology of Semiconductor Devices* and then joined Robert Noyce and Gordon Moore as the third employee of a company called Intel, which did quite well. He was a most admirable man and lived an inspiring life. In 1983 he published a seminal book entitled *High Output Management* [1], the antithesis of the managerialist gibberish plaguing our bookshops. It is a work germane to many disciplines including the practice of medicine.

The message is grounding and could not be clearer: our purpose should be the demonstration of safe, lasting clearance of the symptoms and disease.

We should collaborate with our patients to find solutions. Our reach should be much more than slavish, unreflective adherence to policy. But, it is the patients who must judge whether we succeed. If a patient says she is no better, then we have not achieved our objective. It does not matter what tests say, whether we followed guidelines, what we think or feel; the patient did not get better.

Evolution and its role

It is difficult to make sense of cUTI without a solid understanding of evolution and a good story helps even if it is from another territory. Look at Figure 7.1; it shows a caterpillar sitting on eggs so as to protect them. On reflection, this seems peculiar because the caterpillar is destined to pupate and metamorphose into a butterfly or moth which will then lay the eggs that unsupervised, mature into caterpillars. So, are these really eggs and is the caterpillar nurturing them? The answer is yes; if a predator attacks hoping to devour the eggs the caterpillar will try to fight it off because its brain has been hijacked by a parasite that modifies its behaviour purposefully. The eggs did extrude from the caterpillar. These eggs will hatch larvae which will then start feeding on the caterpillar but they will do so carefully so that the vital organs are preserved; thus, the caterpillar is kept alive to be eaten whilst providing protection and fresh sustenance. The larvae will go through several moults until ready to exit. They will number about eighty. Acting in concert they paralyse the caterpillar and over one hour gnaw their way out of their hapless host, flying away as fully formed parasitoid wasps, leaving the caterpillar a denuded shell. It is truly nasty; Charles Darwin wrote of one family of parasitoids, *Ichneumonidae*:

"I cannot persuade myself that a beneficent and omnipotent God would have designedly created the *Ichneumonidae* with the express intention of their feeding within the living bodies of caterpillars."

Nevertheless, in our world we do encourage this behaviour, using it to control agricultural pests.

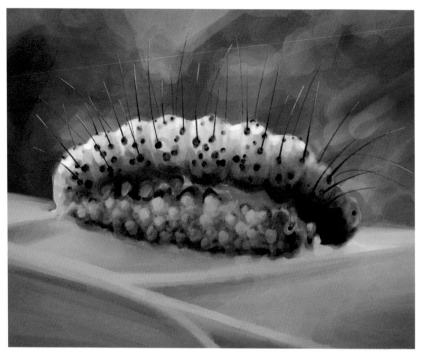

Figure 7.1. The extraordinary sight of a caterpillar nurturing the eggs of a wasp and if predators approach the caterpillar will fight them off. Its brain has been parasitised and its behaviour altered. When the eggs hatch the larvae will eat the caterpillar alive preserving the vital organs until the end. Evolution is immensely inventive of sophisticated mechanisms and we should always remain alert to this potential. The microbial strategies achieving urinary infection are likely to be no less artful and ruthless. *Illustration courtesy of Alex Wilby.*

Whilst this anecdote is fantastic, there are more sophisticated, complicated variations of this mechanism. The inventor is Darwinian evolution, which was described impeccably accurately by one of Darwin's contemporary critics:

"In the theory with which we have to deal, Absolute Ignorance is the artificer; so that we may enunciate as the fundamental principle of the whole system, that, in order to make a perfect and beautiful machine, it is not requisite to know how to make it. This proposition will be found, on careful examination, to express, in condensed form, the essential purport of the Theory, and to express in a few words all Mr. Darwin's meaning; who, by a strange inversion of reasoning, seems to think Absolute Ignorance fully qualified to take the place of Absolute Wisdom in all of the achievements of creative skill." Robert Beverly MacKenzie, 1868.

So why should we bother you with this lurid example of parasitisation in a book on UTI? For a start cUTI is a parasitisation and mightily sophisticated. Evolution is a powerful artificer, which given time, is capable of spectacular feats of invention. The common ancestor of parasitoid wasps evolved approximately 247 million years ago. Bacteria have been around for 3.5 billion years and the urinary bladder for at least 390 million years. We host a polymicrobial bladder microbiome of antibiotic producing bacteria in competition; they are fending off each other, not just our immunity. Bladder-based antibiotic evasion strategies must predate humans by millennia. Do we really consider bacterial UTI so trivial that 3-day treatment is the universal panacea? Do cultures give the answer? Does pyelonephritis only need a 24-hour hospitalisation and a week or two of an oral regimen? Can a guideline nail it? We face a frighteningly sophisticated foe. Do we check for satisfactory recovery? Are there feedback loops? Why do so many sufferers keep returning?

The parasitisation of the caterpillar's brain, forcing defence of the eggs, is like belief memes enslaving our intellects. These force us into views on treatment obstinately held, regardless of evidence. We defend them, using logical fallacies and when all else fails, the emotive and *ad hominem* apologia. These beliefs reflect our needs, be they desperation, hope, wishfulness or greed. Today cognitive psychology has shed much light onto this [2-4].

There is another consideration — evolution is manifestly effective; we can learn from this. It only needs replication, variation, selection and time. During the Pliocene Epoch, we hominids evolved the capacity to think inventively, shorting the millennial wait for serendipitous mutations to solve problems. We can use our intelligence to accelerate evolution of solutions. This is the antithesis of practice authorised by centralised doctrinaire stipulations. One is creative and the other smothering and often wrong.

Fifteen years ago we obeyed the exhortations to conduct a RCT because that was the "only way of proving the case". We were tenacious because we attempted two such RCTs of treatment. They failed because the patients would not agree to the option of a placebo for 6 weeks. Thank heavens for the patients, because we were set to bungle the science badly. We did not know enough to hazard a RCT and our hypothesis was just a bad guess. We had no appreciation of the numerous random events influencing treatment decisions. These include: idiosyncratic drug intolerances, variations in dose requirement, variations in the necessary treatment duration, unpredictable responses to treatment cessation, polymicrobial infections, mixed antibiotic susceptibilities, super-added infections, psychological difficulties and intercurrent illness, and many more random perturbations. Unless you have sorted out these aspects a RCT is a foolish undertaking. This is not a trivial matter; during October 2015, a standard guideline was imposed on the management of our patients and our clinic was closed. At that time one of us had a discussion with a senior academic doctor:

Sen: "You should have done a RCT."
Us: "We tried twice but failed. The hypothesis was naïve anyway."
Sen: "You should have tried harder."

Some weeks later we faced a scrutiny panel made up of important peers. We explained this: the patients were suffering, they had pyuria, negative culture, improved on antibiotics and deteriorated when we stopped them. We asked what would they do instead? After a pause, someone observed: "But your data are not from a RCT". All this is emblematic of a mighty problem: the RCT emperor has eclipsed too much. For example, data from feedback loops, that scrutinise patients' responses, particularly if plotted, are spectacularly revealing. Instead of investing in such reflective practice, we fritter and fuss about protocol compliance because we are deluded that the RCTs and meta-analysis are the last word.

So, let us consider the vexed matter of a RCT. We are qualified for this; we have published peer-reviewed data on 15 RCTs. They are the warp to the basic scientific weft of our centre. We caution against the confident opinions on RCTs voiced by those who have not done these studies. We found little else more humbling for the assured mind than the experiences of trying to do a clinical trial properly.

The randomised controlled trial in perspective

Done with precision for an unbiased estimate of an effect size (not a p-value), the RCT is stellar but has never been the sole arbiter of truth. To be useful a RCT must test a prediction from a coherent, plausible hypothesis, already validated *a priori* by other means. In particular, the target patients and an expected clinically useful effect must be carefully defined. Whether falsifying or verifying, the funders will require confidence in the truth of the hypothesis. Much science, basic and clinical, should predate the RCT. An appropriate outcome measure should be well validated. A RCT does best with clear outcomes such as death (cancer, HIV, COVID-19), easily measured effects (fever, weight, ITU admission) and on a short time frame (acute or rapidly progressive illness). If viable, the RCT is an excellent way of testing Pearl's counterfactuals [5] but it is not the only way.

Given heterogenous patients, from long-tailed distributions, with multiplicity in symptoms and signs, a slow, oscillating response, and many confounders, a RCT is a daunting, sometimes impossible undertaking. We should admit to that and not pretend otherwise.

The MSU culture's simple "positive or negative" is a ubiquitous measure in RCTs of antibiotics for acute infection. This method ignores the symptoms, signs, fluctuations and tenacity of the disease. Much worse, culture as an outcome was never validated and has now been discredited, a false witness. So for this indication, the historical RCT and meta-analysis data look seriously dodgy, which is what the non-RCT data have been shouting about for years.

Rule makers are attracted to the meretricious cleanliness of the "Yes/No" dichotomies. Either you have done a RCT or not; the result was positive or negative; meta-analyses may report odds-ratios of a Yes/No outcome. But we are dealing with the biological complexities of humans. Joint probability distributions encompassing all the evidence, including non-RCT data, are much more honest.

The insistence on the unassailable status of the RCT is forcing some regrettable trends. Hurried, poorly designed, expedient RCTs are more common nowadays and they are bordering on useless. In many cases the sampling frame means that the data are not applicable to the patient in your clinic.

Not being able to do a RCT because of resource constraints is no excuse not to collect evidence to test the validity of an opinion or action. Does anyone bother to test whether guidelines increase the probability of a better patient outcome? We did this, not by doing a RCT, but by using feedback loops and discovered that the guideline practice was making the patients worse. Should we claim they were not getting worse because it wasn't a RCT?

As with granting tests supremacy, we may be inveigled to see RCT data as the last word, rendering all studies upstream irrelevant. In fact, many historical data from the discovery programme are important, despite being snubbed in the trial reports. This promotes a stilted perspective, unenriched by the development science.

Triumphalist parables on RCTs exposing deficiencies in anecdotal and historical practice may have encouraged the attribution of exaggerated powers to the RCT which is then enthroned as the ultimate Panjandrum. We should stop comparing the RCT against such cheap targets and dare to ask, to what extent do RCTs advance on other valid scientific methods and do economic limits license less puritanism. It is not as simple as that; comparative studies have demonstrated that done well, non-RCT clinical science can be just as effective [6, 7]. There is a vast difference between meticulous outcome records contrasted to the recall evidence and traditional lore that the first RCTs refuted.

During the COVID-19 pandemic a question was raised about the safety of going ahead with a football match between Liverpool and Atlético Madrid at Anfield Stadium on 11 March 2020. It was stated that there was no evidence that a gathering of more than 52,000 people would increase the risk of the spread of the Coronavirus. This was technically true if evidence be synonymous with a RCT which was lacking. Given what we knew about the virus and its spread how would probability have judged this? Liverpool lost, so imagine the effect of all that parochial, lachrymose, rhinorrhoea into commiserating embraces.

Clinical evolutionary epistemology

Our cringingly embarrassing failures with the RCTs that we attempted between 2006 and 2011 forced us to reconsider and then admit that we were baffled by these poor patients, desperate for help with their debilitating symptoms. We had no idea what to do. Thus, we resorted to an historical precedent adopted by others when similarly flummoxed. "What do you do when you do not know what to do?" One answer lies in the methods that Alan Turing used to break the Enigma code. Shadowing this approach we used Popperian trial and error elimination [8] and Bayesian inference [9] to work out a process of scientific evolutionary epistemology [10] in order to find a treatment. We installed software that forced feedback loops into our clinical practice. The rules were strict; we had to document our reasons for diagnosis, the justification for treatment and the hypothesis driving any investigation. It forced declarations of our expectations of response and adverse effects. Outcomes were measured, graphed and this information used to reject what failed and to retain what succeeded. Reports of the data from this work are available in the peer-reviewed literature [11-17]. The system was geared to rebuff logical fallacies and *ad hoc*, specious explanation. We were refused the option of using investigations as ploys to defer facing up to unresolved problems. Figure 7.2 echoes Figure 2.1 in depicting the discovery cycle. It is a fact that from 2000 to 2013, the commonest outcome, by a huge margin, found error in our managements. This was an error-assimilation process so that error-trapping and its elimination drove the creative process.

Figure 7.2 identifies the key components of evolution in green: variation, replication and selection, with time omitted. The place of scientific thinking is shown by the arrows of induction, abduction and deduction.

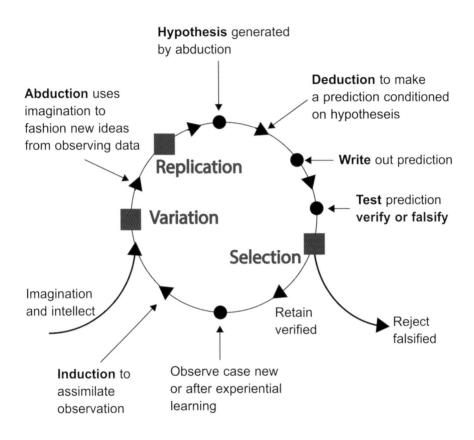

Figure 7.2. Scientific evolutionary epistemology.

Notice that a hypothesis must lead to a written prediction, otherwise its testing will lack purpose and risk random occurrences clouding the picture. As with Micawberisms, a random, unexpected event is most probably erroneous. The evaluation of the prediction will verify or falsify; and what is falsified must be rejected, not retained through sophistry.

The evidence-based medicine (EBM) vernacular may have muddled our understanding of the cycle depicted in ▨ Figure 7.2. Lexicography confuses the meaning of "empiricism". An "empiricist" can be a physician of the ancient classical world who held that treatment should be based on observation rather than theory. Alternatively, it can mean a quack! Sometimes doctors speak of "treating empirically" and this means going by an "educated guess" when empirical evidence is deficient. Thus, to some the empirical methods may be considered anathema as others are scandalised by the notion of trial and error elimination. We have been reported for doing both — reader if you are perplexed, we thank you for your companionship.

The clinical problem

We face a bad situation. There are increasing numbers of patients, the majority female, suffering from chronic, painful lower urinary tract symptoms punctuated by acute flares, akin to an acute cystitis. Those affected often exhibit negative urine culture. Erroneously, the culture result is invoked to dismiss a positive leucocyte esterase dipstick test, despite the specificity of that insensitive test. Too many patients are told that they could not have a UTI and too often they attract the specious diagnosis of "interstitial cystitis", "painful bladder syndrome" or "bladder pain syndrome".

Are the patients diseased?

The evidence that demonstrates the failures of dipsticks and MSU culture does not imply that the patient cluster has UTI; it just reduces the probability that UTI was legitimately excluded. To incriminate UTI we need greater verification. When comparing these patients with normal controls, the corroboration stacks up. Microscopy of a fresh, unstained, unspun urine sample using a haemocytometer reveals pyuria and epithelial shedding that correlates with symptoms [12, 18]. The patients show evidence of elevation in urinary cytokines IL-6, CXCL8, lactoferrin and ATP [19]; these also correlate with symptoms [13, 14, 17]. Advanced culture methods and urinary 16S rRNA microbiome analysis demonstrate increased microbial load with wider species dispersion [17]. Uroepithelial cell exfoliation is increased along with greater microbial parasitisation of the cells [18]; all this despite negative cultures and dipsticks. The peer-reviewed data make UTI the most probable explanation of the symptoms because of those supplemental findings.

It cannot be overstated that our contemporary knowledge is certainly not inadmissible, pending completion of a definitive trial. An egregious disease, appalling suffering and life-changing consequences are not to be dismissed. It is not okay to cling to the interstitial cystitis diagnosis or some other questionable concept until a final trial speaks. We must respond to our patients using the best available evidence even when that set is yet incomplete.

Is there evidence for causation?

Machine learning, and its applications in computational biology, has had a transforming effect on our understanding of causation. Judea Pearl, a major contributor, brings this science to a broader audience in *The Book of Why* [20]. He uses a metaphor; the ladder of causality:

- Correlation.
- Intervention.
- Counterfactual.

The first rung is correlation; whilst not the same as causation, the latter cannot exist without the former. The next rung is intervention; doing something affects the probability of a hypothesis. Pearl invented the "do" operator for the necessary maths (the notation is: P[Hypothesis] | do[Intervention]). The final rung is the assimilation of counterfactuals; what would be the case if a seminal event did not happen? The RCT is a formal method of evaluating a counterfactual, using a placebo group. These steps build the probability of a hypothesis about causation. We found correlations between our patients' symptoms and pathophysiological markers of infection [13, 14]. We intervened by treating with antibiotics; we stopped these treatments routinely to record symptoms relapse. We reported a study of outcomes from the sudden arbitrary cessation of treatment, thus testing the counterfactual [16] and in time we shall finesse this with a RCT.

How we manage the patients

We start with patients who describe chronic painful LUTS, negative urine dipsticks and cultures. Fresh urine microscopy provides pyuria and uroepithelial cell counts. We have a symptom score that is unusually well validated. We have good reason to diagnose a probable infection but have no means of fingering the causative pathogens and describing their antibiotic sensitivities.

The principles are as follows:

- Use the clinical history, symptoms, signs and fresh urine microscopy to make a diagnosis (UTI) [13].
- Prescribe a treatment that, given published evidence, is probably effective for UTI (chose from the set of first-generation, narrow-spectrum, urinary antibiotics and the urinary disinfectant methenamine).
- The choice of treatment must be supported by empirical evidence encouraging belief in a therapeutic potential. Theoretic belief is not an option.
- If the patient describes a partial response, increase the dose within prescribing limits.
- If the patient does not respond change the prescription to another antibiotic of the same set.
- If the patient cannot tolerate the medication change to another antibiotic from the same set.
- When the symptoms, signs and urine microscopy have normalised, stop the treatment.
- If symptoms resurge on cessation, restart the treatment.
- Repeat this process until the treatment may be stopped with impunity.
- Keep meticulous records of all of the actions and use these data to learn and identify best options for future patient management.

This approach combines feedback loops, learning and evolution through reflective clinical practice. It results in a continuous process of renewal, informed by a growing data set. After a long time, well over a decade, a promising protocol thus evolves, which should continue to improve towards a theoretical optimum. Richard Arkwright and John Kay used a similar approach to invent the spinning frame during the 1760s. Indeed, this Enlightenment, empirical science drove the Industrial Revolution. It saddened us that some colleagues were scandalised by these methods and campaigned to stop us, in the interests of "evidence-based medicine"; from its beginnings with such promise of a happy future, this movement has become so badly disfigured by arbitrary regulating, formalisation of process and spurious righteousness. No matter; we now have a treatment protocol, after 20 years treating such patients, suitable for a RCT, and a validated means of managing our patients whilst we await those results.

Now we are placed to describe the approach to assessment and treatment that is current practice in our tertiary centre. The method description and its validation is in the peer-reviewed literature [15, 16].

The patients

The patients of interest suffer from lower urinary tract symptoms likely to include recurrent urinary infections, chronic bladder pain, interstitial cystitis and chronic cystitis. Those presenting to our centre had had their symptoms for an average of 5 years. The average age of the patients is 50 (95% CI 48 to 51), 80% female, 20% male. Most will describe a history of multiple tests and consultations in secondary and/or tertiary care. The story of symptoms despite numerous normal urinalyses is common and most patients believe that doctors think there is nothing wrong with them. The typical investigations that have been used include blood tests, renal tract and pelvic ultrasound scans, CT scans, MRI scans, and urodynamics. Most patients will have undergone cystoscopy, with or without urethral dilation or cystodistension. Bladder biopsies will have revealed various manifestations of chronic cystitis. It is common to report multiple cystoscopies. Other than bladder biopsies, these various investigations will usually have proved negative. A variety of bladder infusion treatments may have been attempted without benefit.

Their previous treatments may include the following list of failed remedies: bladder retraining, fluid management, dietary management, cranberry extracts, D-mannose, various antibiotics including prophylaxis, overactive bladder medications, physiotherapy, urethral dilation, cystodistension, urothelial cautery, botulinum toxin injections, urethral and bladder steroid injections, bladder instillations, pain management, psychological interventions, oestrogens, antihistamines, pentosan polysulfate sodium (Elmiron®), sacral and tibial nerve stimulation, acupuncture, alternative therapies, probiotics, herbal remedies, "urovaccines", low histamine diet, ozone treatment.

The scientific evidence for the efficacy of most of these methods is sparse or zero. In most cases their use is not justified. Why deploy a treatment such as urethral dilation, when it is devoid of evidence of benefit?

The symptoms and signs

The symptoms that we seek are summarised in ▮ Table 7.1 and this set has been thoroughly validated [13].

The voiding symptoms are the most sensitive predictors of a pyuria and in both sexes they are the first to develop and the last to resolve in the event of a UTI. Contrary to common assumption, pain is not the dominant symptom but is secondary to voiding symptoms. Frequency and all the symptoms of an overactive bladder may feature, as may stress incontinence. This fact mandates the careful exclusion of infection when addressing the urinary incontinence clusters.

The signs that we look for are suprapubic tenderness, loin tenderness, urethral tenderness and prostate tenderness. Strange as it may seem, these are yet to be validated in clinical studies so we must own up to acting on assumption.

Table 7.1. The question inventory used in our clinical service presented in the order that we ask. This set has been thoroughly validated through a number of clinical studies and found to be commensurate with biological measures of the pathophysiology. It is important that the questions are dichotomised "Yes or No" without modifying value judgements which would inject considerable inter-operator variability.

Storage symptoms	Stress symptoms	Voiding symptoms	Pain symptoms
1. Urgency	12. Cough sneeze incontinence	20. Hesitancy	27. Suprapubic pain
2. Urge incontinence	13. Exercise incontinence	21. Reduced stream	28. Filling bladder pain
3. Latchkey urgency		22. Intermittent stream	29. Voiding bladder pain
4. Latchkey urge incontinence	14. Laughing incontinence	23. Straining to void	30. Post-void pain
5. Waking urgency	15. Passive incontinence	24. Terminal dribbling	31. Pain relieved by voiding
6. Waking urge incontinence	16. Bending incontinence	25. Post-void dribbling	32. Partial voiding relief
7. Running water urgency	17. Standing incontinence	26. Double voiding	33. No voiding relief
8. Running water urge incontinence	18. Lifting incontinence		34. Loin pain
9. Cold urgency	19. Pre-cough preparation		35. Iliac fossa pain
10. Anxiety urgency			36. Pain radiation to genitals
11. Perimenstrual aggravation			37. Pain radiation to legs
			38. Dysuria
			39. Urethral pain

Special aspects of the clinical history

The pain symptoms may radiate unexpectedly. The legs, arms, and shoulders may feature. Vulval and genital pain are common and some will locate the feeling between the rectum and genitalia. Men describe an unpleasant penile tip pain.

We identify loin pain and tenderness in a significant number who do not describe other features of pyelonephritis and there are no white blood cell casts in the urine. We do not know whether this symptom reflects low-grade renal involvement, pain referral or renal capsule stretch because of increased blood flow through the urinary tissues.

Certain foodstuffs may cause symptom exacerbations; chocolate, coffee, alcohol, spicy foods and acidic foods such as fizzy drinks are common culprits but people vary a great deal in their susceptibility and there is no consistency.

It is notable that sex, smear tests, gynaecological procedures, horse riding, cycling, high-impact exercise, running, swimming and cold can result in acute exacerbations. Air flight can do it as well. We do not know the mechanisms but suspect two options as plausible. One could be physical or chemical stresses acting on an inflamed and already painful urothelium. The other is that perturbation of parasitised urothelial cells results in activation of the dormant microbes which then start dividing, destroy the host cell and break out into the tissues to stimulate an acute inflammatory flare.

Constipation and defaecation can aggravate the symptoms with some experiencing relief from defaecation whilst others have pain persisting for some time afterwards. We assume that pressure effects on the inflamed urogenital tract explain this. Similarly, men may experience pain with ejaculation because of prostatitis and inflammation of the urogenital tract.

The pelvic muscle pain and tension features settle slowly with treatment of infection. There is a tendency for it to select one particular side. Perhaps the cause is protective muscle tension, guarding tender urinary tract tissue.

Voiding dysfunction symptoms seem to be related intimately to urine infection in both sexes. They prove to be the earliest symptoms to present and the last to clear. They feature a reduced stream, intermittency and terminal dribbling sometimes with straining and post-micturition dribbling. We have yet to explain the mechanism but swelling of the urethral tissues from the oedema of an inflammatory reaction is plausible and hesitancy resulting from pain another option.

The symptoms of the overactive bladder including frequency, urgency and urge incontinence may also feature. Strangely, stress urinary incontinence can resolve on treating infection.

We often record systemic symptoms, notable fatigue, brain fog, depression, anxiety and problems with concentration. Nausea and vomiting may feature.

The investigations

The single crucial test is immediate microscopy of a fresh urine sample that is unspun, unstained and mounted in a haemocytometer counting chamber. This is conducted in the clinic at the time of seeing the patient.

Urine (1µl) is loaded into a clean Neubauer haemocytometer counting chamber (Figure 7.3) [21]. This preparation is examined using a x20 objective with a x10 eyepiece (magnification x200). The leucocyte count (wbc/µl) are enumerated by counting cells in five large squares out of nine and multiplying the result by two because the volume of the whole chamber is 0.9µl. If a cell overlaps a dividing line it is counted if the line runs along the top or right side and ignored if the line runs along the bottom or left side. The same method is used to count the uroepithelial cells.

We do not act on the results of a urine culture. The data obtained from such sources are ignored. This will be addressed in greater detail in the coming chapter. A dipstick leucocyte result is interpreted on the understanding that is highly specific but hopelessly insensitive. Nitrite analysis is ignored because it has been so thoroughly discredited.

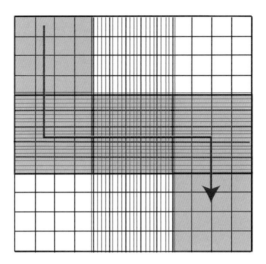

Figure 7.3. Neubauer haemocytometer counting chamber.

The red arrow shows the pattern used to search for and count the cells in the urine sample over five large squares. If the count is low we should count over the entire chamber.

Using graphs

It would be hard to overemphasise the critical importance of using graphs plotting the symptoms score, urinary white blood cell count and uroepithelial cell count over the assessments. As will become clear in subsequent paragraphs the knowledge gleaned from these graphs will:

- Show the direction of travel of a system that changes slowly.
- Prevent misinterpretation of symptom flares.
- Encourage loyalty to the prescription regimen and discourage shuffling of antibiotics.
- Reassure when the symptom response lags.
- Refute suspicions of resistance development.

Other investigations

A renal ultrasound scan if not done already is advisable. A tenacious high pyuria should always alert to stone disease. Persistent haematuria, particularly frank haematuria, requires exclusion of cancer. Men should undergo a rectal examination, if not already done. The PSA is difficult to interpret in the face of cUTI but notably high levels should ring alarm bells.

The treatment regimen

We have published on this regimen and then described data from a crossover study of unplanned cessation of treatment [16]. We are going to describe our current clinic protocol here on the understanding a RCT is pending.

(For those conversant with the causation revolution in A.I., the first published study successfully applied an intervention of Pearl's second rung ["do" operator P(A | do(B = b))] and the second tested the counterfactual of the third rung. So, there is legitimacy in describing our practice now.)

Patients presenting with symptoms but without microscopic pyuria

We do not initiate an antibiotic regime unless there is a pyuria signal. Many patients will attend with the appropriate symptoms but their urinalysis by microscopy proves negative. The commonest reason is that they have been advised to over-imbibe and the urine is dilute. In these circumstances it is better to review and defer treatment until there is a urinary cellular signal to plot. If the symptoms are compelling, methenamine may be used on its own during the interregnum. So, whilst acknowledging a sensitivity less than 100%, we insist on this signpost before starting an antibiotic. If the symptoms are compelling it is still best to re-test and stay with methenamine alone unless a pyuria presents. Methenamine can be effective on its own, albeit with a slow action.

An antibiotic and a disinfectant

We start with an antibiotic and prescribe this alone for 14 days and then add in methenamine. The staggered initiation allows us to detect intolerance and attribute it accurately. This is particularly the case in relation to methenamine which can sometimes cause dysuria when first used. It is an acidic drug capable of aggravating an inflamed urinary tract. This problem may cease to arise when the inflammation has settled down, which should occur in response to the antibiotic. About every 4 weeks we retest it gently by building the dose up, gradually starting with half a tablet a day and backing out if the symptoms return again. As the antibiotic treatment continues, further attempts at restarting methenamine may be made from time to time. Eventually it is likely that the methenamine will be acceptable at full dose at which point we start to experiment with the withdrawal of the antibiotic. The target is to achieve a situation where all is well on methenamine alone and from there to a treatment-free state.

The antibiotic options

The antibiotic selection is made from the set of first-line agents which are tried in the following order based on tolerance first and then efficacy:

- Cefalexin 500mg qid.
- Nitrofurantoin macrocrystals CR 100mg bid.
- Trimethoprim 200mg bid.
- Pivmecillinam 200mg tid.

Cefalexin is a first-generation cephalosporin and should not be confused with the more powerful later-generation agents used for serious infections. 80% of the dose is excreted in the urine so it is useful for urinary infections. It has none of the more significant properties and side effects of the later-generation agents. In terms of safety in long-term use, it is top of our league table and it has the lowest *Clostridium difficile* (*C. diff*) rate of the antibiotics.

Nitrofurantoin has been found to be the drug that achieves the greatest penetration of the urothelial cells and so it gets close to the heart of the pathology. It is absorbed rapidly from the gastrointestinal tract and excreted immediately by the kidneys, thus concentrating where it is needed. Ordinary nitrofurantoin makes people feel sick, but given as macrocrystals this is less of a problem. We should not use nitrofurantoin in anyone with a history of interstitial lung disease. It is important to be alert to the more serious side effects: cough or shortness of breath, paraesthesia or sensory neuropathy. These side effects of nitrofurantoin are rare but they are important because they are responsive to immediate cessation.

Trimethoprim is an old standard although there is a degree of ambient resistance. The efficacy may be enhanced by increasing the dose and our data imply that combining with methenamine is synergistic. Trimethoprim can compete with creatinine for secretion into the renal tubule causing benign elevation of blood creatinine, which may induce misplaced alarm in the unwary.

Pivmecillinam is significantly more expensive. Out of all these agents it has a greater tendency to cause upper gastrointestinal side effects that may exhibit delayed onset after some weeks.

The second-line agents which are deployed uncommonly and reluctantly to address recalcitrant symptoms or multiple intolerances are:

- Amoxicillin 500mg bid.
- Co-amoxiclav 625mg bid.
- Fosfomycin 3g thrice weekly.

It is tempting to think that a short sharp shock of aggressive treatment will sort the situation out well and good. These methods have been tried and found disappointing. The IV regimens in particular are seductive as they can have an immediate dramatic effect on the symptoms, such that we may be persuaded that the problem has been resolved, only to be dismayed by a resurgence within a week or two of cessation of treatment

Figure 7.4 records a salutary experience from our past and which you would never catch us doing again. We were trying to get to grips with an unusually nasty infection and resorting to IV ertapenem regimens of

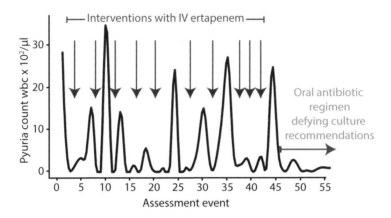

Figure 7.4. Urinary white blood cells by assessment event; data were collected whilst trying to treat a nasty chronic infection. They demonstrate the abject failure of IV regimens.

The graph plots out the urinary pyuria which was particularly high. The patient was certainly sick. The black arrows mark out the interventions with IV ertapenem which achieved a gratifying response that reversed as soon as we stopped. The green horizontal arrow indicates the use of a high-dose oral regimen that was prescribed in contradiction of the microbiological culture isolate sensitivity data.

increasing duration on the understanding that by hitting the infection hard and decisively we should succeed in eradicating it. In fact, each time that we stopped the IV infusions, the infection bounced right back again. Eventually we abandoned the approach, rejected the culture sensitivity data that were encouraging ertapenem and treated with oral co-amoxiclav. We shall discuss how culture sensitivity data may exert an inflationary influence on antibiotic selection in the coming chapter.

The core problem is that the microbes persist inside the cells and in niches where they are protected by biofilms. They are dormant and not dividing and so they are impervious to antibiotic attack. As soon as the IV or powerful regimen is withdrawn these sleepers break out into the spaces that have been cleared and the symptom cycle starts all over again. This problem is germane to the brief hospital admissions for treating pyelonephritis when follow-up after discharge is not done. We are too easily reassured by a gratifying response to an IV infusion and we surmise that the future is rosy. Do we have evidence for such optimism? We need to introduce outcome feedback into the management of these patients.

The treatment process

We seek to establish a first-generation antibiotic regimen that is tolerated and shown to be effective because of an improvement in the symptoms score and in the urine microscopy, without significant side effects.

If we can spot a symptom response, no matter how incomplete, then we tend to advise persistence with the regimen to allow this to grow into something more substantial. The symptoms tend to clear gradually one feature after another with some alterations in quality along the way.

We have made regrettable errors when patients have felt pressure to achieve an effective response because of a pending deadline. The failure of an early resolution has prompted prescription change with detrimental results. It is more often the case that the original prescription was correct and that the shuffling of antibiotics to hurry progress was harmful.

Once the first-line regimen has been established, we add methenamine 1g twice daily and sustain this with the selected antibiotic.

If the patient describes symptoms resurging with the medication trough just before a dose is due or when medication is omitted, it implies an inadequate prescription that should be raised.

We do not expect a linear response and should be averse to over-interpreting the natural fluctuations in the healing process. Symptom flares pepper the history of treatment. A good response may be subverted by an eruption of unpleasant symptoms. In addition, if the patient is recovering, the symptoms can feel more severe than at the outset, despite the microscopic evidence of disease activity being less. Perhaps the diminishing inflammation leaves a supersenstivity in its wake. Many of these acute flares settle without a need to do anything different although some require a temporary dose increase.

The recovery involves a series of oscillations of decreasing amplitude so that graphs of the symptoms and urinary cell counts plot out a damped oscillation of reducing peaks, falling to a full resolution (Figure 7.5). It is important not

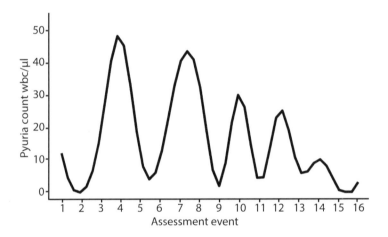

Figure 7.5. A plot of urinary cell counts against assessment dates — a damped oscillation slowly evolves whilst the treatment regimen is administered consistently without changes of prescription.

This record is taken from a 76-year-old woman who presented with a 7-year history of recurrent urinary tract infection which had metamorphosed into chronic bladder pain and lower urinary tract symptoms typical of urinary tract infection. The plot shows a classic damped oscillation and we should confess to being rattled by the early peaks associated with acute flares and in response we did indeed shuffle that antibiotic regimen with poor results. She started on cefalexin and methenamine and stays on the same. We have to be patient and let it oscillate down, changing treatment only if this pattern is disrupted.

to misinterpret the peaks as implying a treatment failure or the development of resistance, which is remarkably rare (*v. infra*). If a graph is maintained, the overall decline in counts will be appreciated, whereas isolated point estimates can mislead. The symptoms behave similarly (Figure 7.6).

It is slow and we are not going to get away with short-duration treatment. 75% of patients are able to start coming off antibiotic treatment within 12

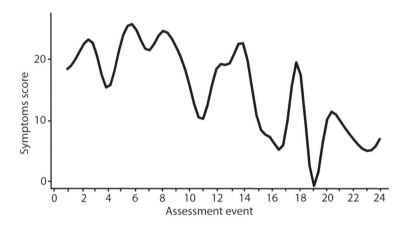

Figure 7.6. Symptoms score by assessment event. The symptoms record of a young adult under treatment having spent her childhood plagued by lower urinary tract symptoms. She relates her story in Chapter 10.

This symptom score has been thoroughly validated. The data are from a young woman who presented to us when aged 20. Her story is related in her letter to the Royal College of Paediatrics and Child Health that is reproduced in the chapter on children. The oscillations of decreasing amplitude are well shown. The point is that you should not assume that because the symptoms have come down, it is all over and do not think that exacerbations mean treatment failure or resistance. They are expected trials along the road to recovery. Note how long it takes to achieve progress. In this case there was an excessively long story and the treatment regimen had to be maintained for a long time, over several years. This plot was a godsend because the powerful influence of recall bias meant that she struggled to assess how she was doing. The damped oscillation instilled some fortitude over the regimen and it paid off although there is some way to go yet.

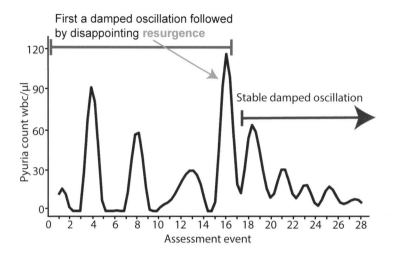

Figure 7.7. Urinary white blood cells by assessment event — we bungled this management by withdrawing antibiotic treatment prematurely and this resulted in a nasty resurgence so that we had to achieve another damped oscillation.

This was a worrying case — a 62-year-old woman with a lifelong history of recurrent urinary tract infections that had evolved into a chronic painful disease with life-changing consequences. We achieved on damped oscillation but she suffered a nasty relapse that required some struggle to get her back to the healing pattern.

months. Our mean treatment length is about 383 days but there is a wide variance (sd=347; 95% CI=337-428). This fact alone compels an insistence on the old, first-generation, narrower-spectrum agents.

The course may not be plain sailing. Sometimes it can be difficult to achieve the much-desired damped oscillation. Figure 7.7 is from a patient who had a tough time of it until we eventually secured the response we were seeking. Figure 7.8 is an alarming chaotic response that is a result of unreliable compliance with the medication regimen. The difficulty is that success depends on patience, perseverance and dogged persistence; flicking on and off treatment is counterproductive.

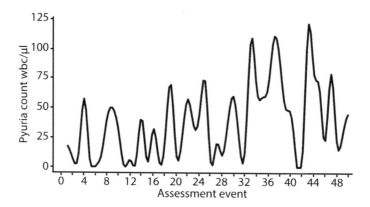

Figure 7.8. Urinary white blood cells by assessment event — a most unsuccessful case that shows a chaotic record. We contributed to this by agreeing to reduce or stop treatment on request. Compliance and dogged persistence are most important.

This disturbing result is a consequence of poor compliance with the medication being used intermittently in response to symptoms. The worry is that the area under the curve is increasing which is the opposite of what we should wish. The signs of progress at the end of this sequence was in the end confounded by a decision to seek natural remedies. At this time we have no options other than strict perseverance; compliance is a major concern because inconsistency is dangerous. So, in the clinic, we are developing the use of lateral flow immunochromatographic assays for checking the urine for the prescribed antibiotics.

There are some remarkably fortunate persons who achieve a rapid onset and gratifying response. Figure 7.9 illustrates one such case which features a critically damped oscillation and an uninterpreted recovery without acute flares to stumble through. Our surveillance data from 7000 patients treated shows that 75% of responses are damped oscillations, 15% critically damped and 10% experiencing a more chequered path as in Figure 7.7. Fortunately, Figure 7.8 is remarkably rare and will be generated in the face of multiple intolerances and compliance difficulties.

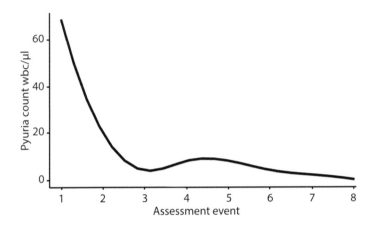

Figure 7.9. Urinary white blood cells by assessment event — the glorious and unusual (15%) critically damped oscillation; there should be dancing in the street.

The critically damped oscillation is always most welcome because it is so decisive. The patient does not have to go through the oscillations and acute flares on the road to recovery. We do not know why this happens in some nor what the mechanism might be. We certainly hope to discover this one day.

If an acute flare proves egregious or persistent an intervention is justified. We double the dose of the antibiotic and sometimes the methenamine. If the patient has been on an effective regimen, we should be reluctant to change it because it will usually reassert itself. We should not consider altering the prescription without doing a urinalysis and seeing change in the urinary inflammatory signal that would justify such a regrettable move. Most of the time the wisest course is to wait for the flare to settle. It is most likely to be an inconvenient, natural fluctuation in the course of the disease resolution.

Once the symptoms and urinalysis show a damped oscillation, we follow this down to a flat baseline. However, we insist on periodic checks on efficacy through brief treatment stops which if resulting in symptom resurgence, confirm the medication need. Some patients are bound to forget their medication or reduce off it for some reason. This is an experiential opportunity to check on symptoms rebound — a useful alternative to a deliberate cessation. When the symptoms and the urinary microscopy have normalised, we start a sequence of trials without antibiotic, repeating until a successful withdrawal be achieved.

If a symptom response proves partial with a lingering sense of something going on in the background, the antibiotic should be taken up to the highest permitted and tolerated dose. If that fails, the efficacy of the antibiotic should be checked by a short-lived stop/start experiment. If this proves positive the antibiotic should be reintroduced at a standard dose and a suitable companion antibiotic added in. It is our suspicion that the need to combine agents has less to do with resistance and is more a reflection of the fact that these infections require high doses to achieve a response.

The key guidance comes from the graphs of the urinalysis and symptoms. If there is a downward trend in these graphs, we should stick with the regimen despite the fluctuations.

Intolerance is the commonest reason for altering the prescription and in some patients, this can require much shuffling to find an effective, tolerated regimen. This can result in considerable multiplicity at the outset.

We used to be persuaded into a prescription change, because progress seemed to disappoint, causing an acute reactive, symptom surge and a heedful return to the previous regimen.

Our plan is to achieve a situation where the patient is symptom-free, having reduced off the antibiotic and is taking methenamine on its own. The methenamine may be discontinued at a time when the patient feels free of symptoms, controlled and safe to do this.

Feedback loops

Our opinions are fickle things so we need negative feedback to correct for this, but the quality of this information is equally important.

The COVID-19 pandemic has generated some salutary lessons for us. We ceased to be able to obtain data from the microscopic urinalysis and so had to manage on symptoms. Our email service was a heavily used feedback loop and provided surveillance that picked up patients whose treatment needed correction. Some messages described alarming symptom exacerbation and which caused us to make changes. From this a cycle of ill-advised prescription shuffling then evolved. On restarting urinalysis, we realised the written symptom descriptions were of the moment, reacting to upsetting oscillations during a slow but otherwise encouraging response. The language of the messages emphasised the distress at the time whereas the treatment had nevertheless been effective. Urinalysis graphs are needed to reassure patients and clinicians of progress when symptoms are slow to resolve, with acute flares along the way. Unless side effects occur, treatment changes should always be informed by microscopy, which commonly advises patience.

The antibiotics in action

The action of antibiotics in relation to urinary tract infection is not as simple as the killing of delinquent microbes. The microbiome of the bladder is too complicated for such a neat tale. An antibiotic may result in a symptom response, an exacerbation of symptoms or a response followed by a flare in symptoms. In the same vein, stopping an antibiotic may result in a symptom flare but also an improvement. We only wish the latter were more common.

The bladder in health and disease is colonised by many different microbes. An antibiotic causes the demise of a proportion of the resident species. That offers an opportunity for others that might not be susceptible to the treatment agent, to colonise the vacated space. Usually this is achieved by friendly bugs that are not at all pathogenic and no symptoms result. Less commonly, a pathological species occupies the niche and starts to thrive, thus causing symptoms. If the patient is at home in their own environment, probability favours the triumph of the more friendly microbes and the abatement of symptoms. Thus, in the face of a flare, it is always worth delaying a while to see if it all settles down.

A lifelong habit of prevention

Once off antibiotics we ask patients to have a ready supply of antibiotics available to start on the first hint of a recurrence of cystitis. Such acute attacks should clear rapidly if treated promptly. The antibiotic should be taken in full dose until the symptoms have settled. This tends to take between 1 and 7 days. The science implies that immediate effective treatment diminishes the risk of return to a lingering chronic disease. The key is to start the antibiotics at the first hint of trouble. Patients may delay because of doubt; it is better to be assertive and safe.

The tetracycline/macrolide responsive group

We must address a subset of patients — 15% of our case load. They present an intriguing story but it is under-researched and we have much validation work to do. We have described evolutionary epistemology earlier and this subset was thrown up in the system that we were operating. Bayesian statisticians, analysing our data independently, identified a cluster of patients that separated out from the rest. Coincidentally we had identified the same subset because their treatment pathway had evolved differently to the larger 80% of our patients. Their characteristics tend to be as follows, although this is far from absolute and we have much more to learn:

- The symptom complex features pain particularly centred on the urethra and vagina and was associated with dyspareunia.
- The urethral pain was notably worse after micturition.
- Voiding symptoms of hesitancy, reduced stream and terminal dribbling were prominent, particularly during an acute flare.
- Symptom exacerbations were associated with bowel loading and/or defaecation.

- Sex, vaginal examination and other pelvic procedures were painful and aggravated symptoms.
- Other symptoms included pain radiating down the legs and into the right and left iliac fossa.
- There was no urethral discharge and sexually transmitted disease screens were negative.
- Men were included in the cluster with pain aggravated by ejaculation and bowel activity. They had all been seen by urologists and considered to suffer from chronic prostatitis.
- The microscopic urinalysis showed a low white blood cell count, typically <10 wbc/µl but an elevated urothelial cell count.
- Urine cultures invariably showed no growth.
- The clinical progress was typically protracted with a slow gradual response to treatment with progress being at time almost imperceptible.

Serendipitous effects noted from treatments for other infections caused us to gravitate to treat these patients with macrolides or tetracyclines, sometimes combined [22]. We used these with methenamine, when this could be tolerated by the urethra. We monitored the symptoms for benefit without side effects. Given a response, we tested this by stopping treatment. We then built up a regimen for a maximum benefit with tolerance. Once this was achieved we tested again by cessation. We continued treatment plotting the outcomes and at intervals repeated trials without medication. Thus, we learned that these patients take so long to recover and manage off treatment.

These findings must undergo further trials including a RCT; some searching microbiological studies must explain what is happening. Tetracyclines and macrolides have anti-inflammatory properties, but we have been unable to get non-steroidal anti-inflammatories to work here.

With many thanks to our patient P. O'Grady in Ireland we reproduce here the symptoms chart of one patient in treatment with this method (Figure 7.10). It is the diminishing areas under the curves that tell the story.

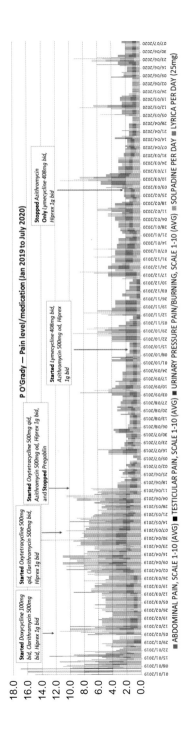

Figure 7.10. The symptoms analysis from a 53-year-old man treated with a combination of lymecycline and azithromycin. Note the oscillations and amplitude decline.

Fluid intake

We are all exposed to the evidence-free advice to drink a great deal in order to wash through the urinary tract. We think that this is wrong. It is best to be governed by thirst; there is nothing better than that. The body's ability to judge how much fluid you need is one of the most perfectly balanced and accurate physiological mechanisms in creation. Our concern is that the increased urine output dilutes the natural antibodies in the urine and additionally aggravates overactive bladder symptoms. If someone is on treatment for UTI, the increased fluid intake will dilute the antibiotic in the urine to ineffective levels.

A salient consequence of the high fluid intakes is that they dilute all pathological signals out of the urine. If a urinalysis is positive and you advise increasing fluid intake, the diluted urine will test negative; bingo! We done wonders!

Oestrogens

Most patients have been exposed to oestrogens before attending us. They have been the subject of numerous clinical trials and it would seem that topical oestrogens, but not systemic HRT, may have a small effect on reducing the number of acute flares [23, 24]. They do not suit everyone so their prescription must use trial and error elimination.

Analgesia

The patients report that pain killers are not particularly effective for the symptoms of urinary tract infection. Ibuprofen at 400mg three times a day can be used as the first option and this can be enhanced by taking paracetamol with the ibuprofen at 1g three times a day. Antihistamines may have analgesic properties [25]. The persistent pain associated with chronic cystitis or urethritis is best managed by using amitriptyline in a small dose of 25mg nocte. Gabapentin or pregabalin are additional options when amitriptyline disappoints [26]. If methenamine is not being used, acute urethral dysuria can be helped by an alkalising agent obtained from the local pharmacy. The opioids do not seem to be effective for chronic pain of cUTI symptoms and should be avoided. Some of our patients present on narcotic analgesics. Our reading is that a withdrawal programme must be instituted from the beginning [27]. It is troubling that their use is condoned in some IC literature.

The dye phenazopyridine (Baridium, Pyridium, Azo) has some local analgesic effects on the bladder mucosa. It causes a vivid colour change in urine, typically to a dark orange to reddish colour. Azo dyes, used in textiles, printing, and plastic manufacturing, were found to cause bladder cancer. Phenazopyridine has not been shown to do this in humans whilst animal studies suggest a carcinogenic potential.

Candida

We are keen to manage thrush infections with topical treatment if possible.

If we see a marked rise in the pyuria without commensurate symptoms, we are most suspicious of vaginal Candida and questioning will often illicit the symptoms. This is important to recognise, otherwise you may be tempted to treat on the assumption of a bacterial infection exacerbation.

Be alert to oral and oesophageal Candida infections which are a risk with long-term use of antibiotics.

It is worth trying to avoid pharmaceutical fungicides as well by using simpler approaches to treatment or prevention.

Boric acid vaginal pessaries are a coherent option when dealing with troublesome Candida. They can be purchased easily without a prescription and they are worth trying.

Unless the vaginal epithelium is severely excoriated, only a limited amount of boric acid is systemically absorbed; it does not pose a threat to a foetus. Treatment is boric acid 600mg intravaginally per night for 14 consecutive nights. It can then be used once or twice weekly as prevention and that is its more important function.

The pharmacists stock various vaginal acidifying products that work on the same principle.

If a fungicide is needed, then a topical application is a preferred option but it should always be followed by prevention.

Gastrointestinal considerations

We are worried about the effect of protracted antibiotic treatment on the gut flora. The evidence for the use of probiotics is not there. We base our advice on applying selection pressure by changing the bacterial feeding substrate that enters the colon. So a diet rich in fruit, vegetables, aimed at increasing fibre with the use of resistant starch, is an option.

Resistant starch is not fully broken down and absorbed. Intestinal bacteria feed on this and thrive. The starch of grains, seeds and legumes are bound to the fibrous cell walls. The crystalline structure of starch in potatoes and bananas resists digestion. If you cook potatoes, rice and pasta and then let them cool they will form resistant retrograded starch.

If a probiotic is really sought, we tend to point our patients at kefir because it saves them spending out on expensive nonsense.

There is no diet that protects against UTI other than that of a healthy lifestyle which is just good for systemic wellbeing. There are fad diets which seem to promote much penance for no gain.

There are no data to suggest that inflammatory bowel disease or irritable bowel disease are associated with chronic UTI. The hypothesis of the intestinal origin of UTI has encouraged the expectation of an association. The molecular methods for species identification of bacteria will now allow us to unravel the mystery of whether UTI comes from the bowel or not. We do not know.

Evolution is always parsimonious so it would seem more probable for microbe species to evolve to colonise the bowel or the bladder but not both, although this is by no means certain. Modern 16S rRNA next generation sequencing analysis should allow us to get a better understanding of this matter. Early indicators are that the species are divergent [28].

Constipation and defaecation can aggravate the symptoms of cystitis because of the pressure effects on an inflamed and painful bladder.

Adverse effects

The side effects of these treatments and their interactions with concomitant medication are available on-line. Because these regimens are protracted, careful attention to these data is so important. We should like to emphasise some particular concerns.

There is a risk of *C. diff* infection, and diarrhoea should provoke an immediate treatment cessation until this settles. Cefalexin and nitrofurantoin have notably low incidences of this complication [29]. When taking nitrofurantoin there should be no cough or shortness of breath, and no paraesthesia or pins and needles. These symptoms may presage rare but serious adversity and vigilance is required because cessation reliably avoids harm. Cefalexin may cause psychological side effects, notably depression and anxiety. Pins and needles, paraesthesia, itching or burning may be experienced with the use of many different antibiotics. In most cases these symptoms are not due to a peripheral neuropathy. They are dose-dependent and respond to cessation or dose reduction. We see extremity pins and needles, but not peripheral neuropathy, with higher-dose penicillins, cefalexin and trimethoprim. The following UTI antibiotics are associated with peripheral neuropathy: nitrofurantoin, quinolones, sulphonamides, penicillins.

To our knowledge, the only serious adverse event (Common Terminology Criteria for Adverse Events — CTCAE Grade 3) was an eosinophilic pneumonitis associated with the use of nitrofurantoin. A patient with severe LUTS, only ameliorated by nitrofurantoin, was exposed intermittently to the drug over 8 years, with numerous attempts at cessation and use of alternatives. She developed a sudden eosinophilic pneumonitis with some fibrosis. She made an excellent recovery from the pneumonitis.

We are aware of a possible case of nitrofurantoin-related pulmonary disease in a quondam patient failing follow-up. She was on an automatic prescription from her primary care centre.

We favour cefalexin over nitrofurantoin and will seek an alternative to the nitrofurantoin once used for 6 months.

Between 2009 and 2020 we recorded 11 cases of *C. diff* infections out of 5020 (0.2%) patients treated.

660 (13%) patients experienced side effects, the commonest problems being gastrointestinal, skin lesions and dose-related paraesthesia.

We address the problem of AMR in a separate chapter — Chapter 8.

There is a paradox in that 11 CTCAEs were generated when a guideline was imposed on the management of our patients, it being justified on the grounds of safety.

Acute cystitis

Chronic UTI and bladder pain has been our research interest. We should address acute cystitis and explain what we do given an evidence deficiency. There are numerous RCTs on the treatment of UTI with consequent guidelines recommending 3-day antibiotic courses followed by culture-centred diagnosis and prescribing [30-32]. These studies used culture, now discredited, and fail to address the 25% to 35% failure rates [33], making the guidelines anachronistic.

We base our method on published science used to abduct an approach using probability, pending essential clinical trial data. We do have evidence that given acute cystitis, a 3-day full-dose course of a first-generation, narrow-spectrum urinary antibiotic will deal with 65% to 75% of cases. The science compels a full infection clearance to avoid lasting intracellular parasitisation. We use the symptom score and microscopic urinary white blood cell counts. The latter data aid diagnosis but may not exclude. They are most valued to monitor progress using a graph; something that we find indispensable:

- A patient presents with symptoms of acute UTI.
- Collect a symptoms score as above, and record suprapubic and loin tenderness.
- A urine dipstick is not sensitive but if positive, a future test may show improvement and thus validate the treatment.
- If available, achieve a urinary microscopic white blood cell count.
- Prescribe a full-dose course of nitrofurantoin or trimethoprim or pivmecillinam (we hold back cefalexin for cUTI).
- If patients sense a response to the antibiotic it is sustained until all symptoms have cleared.
- If a patient does not sense a shift of symptoms in the next 48 hours, go back to step 1, whilst graphing data.
- If a patient responds but relapses after antibiotic cessation, restart and repeat a trial without treatment once the symptoms have cleared. Repeat this until full resolution.

This protocol is similar to our approach to cUTI with shorter intervals. We plot the progress on charts and ensure full symptoms clearance. This is a provisional protocol; some may interpret the available data differently; hopefully others will do the clinical trials.

Voiding dysfunction and its rituals

We have addressed voiding symptoms at several points because they are important. They are consistently found to cluster in both genders in association with bacterial cystitis [13, 15, 34] and to improve on treatment of the

189

infection. It is plausible that infection causes the voiding problem and not vice versa. We have published data that demonstrates that avoiding intermittent catheterisation where commonly applied saw no increase in infection or adversity [35]. It may be that in some cases intermittent self-catheterisation is meddlesome. Inflammation and swelling of the urethra and sphincter with similar effects on the bladder could all compromise voiding. It would seem wise to clear infection first and then revisit concerns about voiding, unless upper tracts are suffering.

For the same reasons we do not advise our patients to adopt voiding rituals in order to clear the bladder. There is no evidence for a beneficial effect; it is likely to be difficult, uncomfortable, worrisome and achieves no gain.

Similarly, hygiene rituals such as how you wipe and how you pee have no substance. Some persons crave proffering, breathy advice on how we should live our lives to avoid UTI. Large chunks of this verbiage draws on cherished myth and little substance: drink buckets of water; fatten up on cranberry juice; wipe from front to back; empty after intercourse; have sex upended; muddle with your hormones; wear calico knickers. Instead, try hiring a shaman to cast spells. If we do not really know, why should we advise? We can do no better than pursue an uncomplicated, ordinary healthy lifestyle.

Pregnancy

In 1960 Edward Kass [36] published a remarkable study of pregnancy. Pregnant women with positive urine culture ($\geq 10^5$ cfu/ml) were divided into two groups. One was treated with sulfamethoxypyridazine for the duration to term and the others were given placebo. Of mothers in the placebo group, 20/48 (41.7%) developed pyelonephritis in the last trimester or 3 months post-partum, but in the treatment group none developed pyelonephritis (0/40 — 0%). Another study in the same vein similarly reported prevention of pyelonephritis by treating bacteriuria in pregnancy [37]. Since then asymptomatic bacteriuria has been treated in pregnancy but not for the duration of the pregnancy.

Pyelonephritis in pregnancy is serious and may be associated with death and severe maternal morbidity including sepsis and acute respiratory, renal and cardiac failure, pre-eclampsia, miscarriage, preterm birth, small babies.

Recently a Dutch study found that whilst asymptomatic bacteriuria in pregnancy is associated with pyelonephritis, the absolute risk for untreated asymptomatic bacteriuria is low [38]. The authors pointed out that the data supporting the prescription of antibiotics for asymptomatic bacteriuria was generated 60 years ago when clinical scientific and obstetric practices were different. Kass used nutrient agar whereas today we use selective chromogenic agar. Jane Currie in her PhD [39] work finds modern antenatal clinics populated by women different to Kass' samples. Kass was focused on the culture method; he studied an enriched sample at particular risk [36] because the pyelonephritis rate untreated was 42%, so different to the Dutch samples [38]. The question is how to identify that subset?

We must also confront the fact of the discovery of the deficiencies of urine culture. How did Kass' pregnant women differ from ours? Should we be screening for asymptomatic bacteriuria or exploring alternative ways of identifying those at greater risk?

This is a worrying problem. Microscopic pyuria is our best marker of UTI but we do not know whether to treat on pyuria without a positive culture in pregnancy. Our service does so, but when managing women with a history of cUTI associated with miscarriage or infertility. We do not know if this is the correct thing to do; that is a big concern. Unravelling this is going to demand some careful prospective work but it is much needed. Urinary tract infection remains an important risk factor for spontaneous preterm birth in the developing world [40].

Figure 7.11 illustrates the case of a 35-year-old woman who presented to us with only a 12-week history of symptoms of chronic UTI which followed an acute UTI that was managed under standard guidelines. Getting this infection under control was a struggle and she ended up on cefalexin, co-amoxiclav and methenamine. This proved the only means of achieving the damped oscillation that fell gradually along with her symptoms to resolution. She then became pregnant and the rise in the urothelial cell count reflects this.

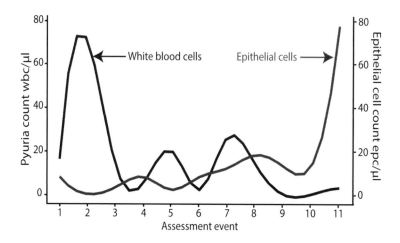

Figure 7.11. Urinary white blood cells and epithelial cells by assessment event — this patient was seeking pregnancy. We achieved a damped oscillation with a rogue peak and then she became pregnant as demonstrated by the epithelial cell count rise typical of normal pregnancy.

These data are from a 35-year old woman who ended up with a cUTI following guideline management. Whilst she presented to us early we had a struggle to get to grips with the infection. We see a second visit pyuria rise quite often and have yet to explain it. In this case we had to use a high-dose combination antibiotic regimen to achieve a response. Once the infection is brought under control many of these women find that they can at last become pregnant. In this case the pregnancy is indicated by the rise in the urothelial cell count which is a feature of normal pregnancy.

The role of stress minus Freud

The relationship with stress or fatigue of any kind is an important physiological association. It is particularly relevant given that these chronic urinary tract infections are invariably caused by bacterial parasitisation of the urothelial cells. These microbes live in rather congenial circumstances with these cells and for most of the time they do not seem active; they are in an otiose state. However, the evolutionary sophistication is remarkable and they can detect higher levels of stress hormones in their host. They use this as a signal to start dividing vigorously, they then burst out of their captured cells and swim off to invade fresh cells whilst the host is under the weather. It is iniquitous.

Patient support

If suffering from a chronic disease it is important to interact with others who are experiencing the same. We notice that people who remain isolated do much less well. Being locked into a personal, idiosyncratic understanding of the disease may be unhelpful. People benefit from the influence of others' perspectives although it is far from obvious until we experience this.

Electronic communications, the internet and social media provide sources of such help which comes through peer groups running mutual support organisations. There are some good ones that are worth exploring. There are chatrooms, advice provision, information libraries and Facebook forums. Here are some useful contacts detailed below*:

Chronic Urinary Tract Infection Campaign (CUTIC)

CUTIC is a UK patient advocacy not-for-profit organisation campaigning for wider recognition of chronic UTI with medical, research and national health care providers. CUTIC runs Facebook support groups which include a women only group, a mixed gender group and a group for parents with children suffering from chronic UTI.

CUTIC'S campaign and day-to-day support websites are detailed below:

cutic.co.uk
chronicutiinfo.com

---

*   The website links provided in this list are not intended to provide an endorsement, approval, recommendation or preference by the author and publisher.

Chronic UTI Women's Support Group
www.facebook.com/groups/chronicUTI

Men & Women's Chronic UTI Support Group
www.facebook.com/groups/1387071144956603

CUTIC-LUTS Children's Group (a private support group for parents)
www.facebook.com/groups/1439446326088527

There is the **Embedded/Chronic UTI Support Group** which is a particularly lively and vociferous option if that appeals. It can be contacted at:

www.facebook.com/groups/ChronicUTISupportGroup

Another option is **Bladder Health UK** which also has a lively forum:

bladderhealthuk.org
www.facebook.com/groups/ICBPSSupportGroup

For those who are living in the Antipodes you are fortunate in having the organisation **Chronic UTI Australia** which is a most impressive, cerebral patient support source:

www.chronicutiaustralia.org.au
www.facebook.com/ChronicUTIAus

There is also the **Chronic and Recurrent UTI Chat Group** (Australia and New Zealand):

www.facebook.com/groups/325213191284414

In the USA, there is **Live UTI free**, which garners accolades from their constituency:

liveutifree.com/About

These groups have different personalities and contrasting approaches. It is worth exploring them to see which fits your preferences.

Social media has its problems. Look at the influence of the anti-vaxxers. There are similar lobbies in the IC and bladder pain environs. They hold implacable opinions on rightful policy, regardless of the science. Contradicting them is a reckless enterprise. If you choose to, expect a torrent of *ad hominem* invective spiced with emotive solipsisms. We consider it best just to apologise for our existence.

Some of the interstitial cystitis sites are less appealing. They seem to be managed by time lords from a bygone age. They are deaf, even hostile to the new science and unreconcilable to the possibility that infection could be a big player. There is too much quackery promoted and some of them are flogging snake oils to the desperate and vulnerable. It can be mightily ugly.

Be cautious of those sites that have links to industry or are supported by commercial sponsorship. They have serious conflicts of interest and a tendency to bang the drum for their sponsors in contradiction to the science.

The future

We think that our protocol is a temporary solution; we need a more sophisticated strategy. Hopefully, research should enlighten our future. The problem of causation must be addressed but conscientiously. Rushing to attribute properties to new methods without evidence is a foolish repetition of the sins of the past. We must find a more expedient method for clinic microscopy. We need to understand better the aftermath of acute cystitis and pyelonephritis. Our grasp of the relevant immunology requires attention. New drugs, which like methenamine, alter urine chemistry to influence urinary ecology, must be preferable to antibiotics. Such options would be so helpful for the elderly.

It is probable that the greatest good will come from a rediscovery of the older ways of using the clinical history, symptoms and signs to inform a coherent differential diagnosis that justifies a few pertinent investigations interpreted with deciding reference to the prior information. We are going to have to own up to the overbearing silliness of some of the guidelines, which have orchestrated pandemonium in the infected bladder.

References

1.   Grove AS. *High output management*, 2nd ed. New York: Vintage; 1995.

2.   Tavris C, Aronson E. *Mistakes were made (but not by me): why we justify foolish beliefs, bad decisions, and hurtful acts*, 1st ed. Orlando, Fla.: Harcourt; 2007.

3.   Shermer M. *The believing brain: from ghosts and gods to politics and conspiracies — how we construct beliefs and reinforce them as truths*, 1st ed. New York: Times Books; 2011: xii, 385.

4.   Syed M. *Black box thinking: why most people never learn from their mistakes — but some do*. New York: Portfolio/Penguin; 2015: xi, 322.

5.   Pearl J. *Probabilistic reasoning in intelligent systems*. San Francisco: Morgan and Kaufman; 2011.

6.   Benson K, Hartz AJ. A comparison of observational studies and randomized, controlled trials. *N Engl J Med* 2000; 342(25): 1878-86.

7.   Frieden TR. Evidence for health decision making — beyond randomized, controlled trials. *N Engl J Med* 2017; 377(5): 465-75.

8.   Popper K. *Objective knowledge, an evolutionary approach*. Oxford: Oxford University Press; 1973.

9.   Herrle SR, Corbett EC, Jr., Fagan MJ, *et al.* Bayes' theorem and the physical examination: probability assessment and diagnostic decision making. *Acad Med* 2011; 86(5): 618-27.

10. Gontier N. Evolutionary epistemology as a scientific method: a new look upon the units and levels of evolution debate. *Theory Biosci = Theor den Biowissenschaften* 2010; 129(2-3): 167-82.

11. Khasriya R, Sathiananthamoorthy S, Ismail S, *et al.* Spectrum of bacterial colonization associated with urothelial cells from patients with chronic lower urinary tract symptoms. *J Clin Microbiol* 2013; 51(7): 2054-62.

12. Kupelian AS, Horsley H, Khasriya R, *et al.* Discrediting microscopic pyuria and leucocyte esterase as diagnostic surrogates for infection in patients with lower urinary tract symptoms: results from a clinical and laboratory evaluation. *BJU Int* 2013; 112(2): 231-8.

13. Khasriya R, Barcella W, De Iorio M, *et al.* Lower urinary tract symptoms that predict microscopic pyuria. *Int Urogynecol J* 2018; 29(7): 1019-28.

14. Gill K, Kang R, Sathiananthamoorthy S, *et al.* A blinded observational cohort study of the microbiological ecology associated with pyuria and overactive bladder symptoms. *Int Urogynecol J* 2018; 29(10): 1493-500.

15. Swamy S, Barcella W, De Iorio M, *et al.* Recalcitrant chronic bladder pain and recurrent cystitis but negative urinalysis: what should we do? *Int Urogynecol J* 2018; 29(7): 1035-43.

16. Swamy S, Kupelian AS, Khasriya R, *et al.* Cross-over data supporting long-term antibiotic treatment in patients with painful lower urinary tract symptoms, pyuria and negative urinalysis. *Int Urogynecol J* 2019; 30(3): 409-14.

17. Sathiananthamoorthy S, Malone-Lee J, Gill K, *et al.* Reassessment of routine midstream culture in diagnosis of urinary tract infection. *J Clin Microbiol* 2019; 57(3): 01452-18.

18. Horsley H, Malone-Lee J, Holland D, *et al. Enterococcus faecalis* subverts and invades the host urothelium in patients with chronic urinary tract infection. *PloS One* 2013; 8(12): e83637.

19. Gill K, Horsley H, Kupelian AS, *et al.* Urinary ATP as an indicator of infection and inflammation of the urinary tract in patients with lower urinary tract symptoms. *BMC Urol* 2015; 15: 7.

20. Pearl J, Mackenzie D. *The book of why: the new science of cause and effect.* London: Allen Lane; 2018.

21. McGinley M, Wong LL, McBride JH, Rodgerson DO. Comparison of various methods for the enumeration of blood cells in urine. *J Clin Lab Anal* 1992; 6(6): 359-61.

22. Perletti G, Marras E, Wagenlehner FM, Magri V. Antimicrobial therapy for chronic bacterial prostatitis. *Cochrane Database Syst Rev* 2013; 8: CD009071.

23. Perrotta C, Aznar M, Mejia R, *et al.* Oestrogens for preventing recurrent urinary tract infection in postmenopausal women. *Cochrane Database Syst Rev* 2008; 2: CD005131.

24. Chen YY, Su TH, Lau HH. Estrogen for the prevention of recurrent urinary tract infections in postmenopausal women: a meta-analysis of randomized controlled trials. *Int Urogynecol J* 2020; doi: 10.1007/s00192-020-04397-z.

25. Raffa RB. Antihistamines as analgesics. *J Clin Pharm Ther* 2001; 26(2): 81-5.

26. Wood H, Dickman A, Star A, Boland JW. Updates in palliative care — overview and recent advancements in the pharmacological management of cancer pain. *Clin Med (Lond)* 2018; 18(1): 17-22.

27. Psaty BM, Merrill JO. Addressing the opioid epidemic — opportunities in the postmarketing setting. *N Engl J Med* 2017; 376(16): 1502-4.

28. Adebayo AS, Ackermann G, Bowyer RCE, *et al.* The urinary tract microbiome in older women exhibits host genetic and environmental influences. *Cell Host Microbe* 2020; 28(2): 298-305.

29. Brown KA, Khanafer N, Daneman N, Fisman DN. Meta-analysis of antibiotics and the risk of community-associated *Clostridium difficile* infection. *Antimicrob Agents Chemother* 2013; 57(5): 2326-32.

30. Anger J, Lee U, Ackerman AL, *et al.* Recurrent uncomplicated urinary tract infections in women: AUA/CUA/SUFU guideline. *J Urol* 2019; 202(2): 282-9.

31. NICE. Urinary tract infection (lower) — women. London: National Institute for Health and Care Excellence, 2014. Available from: http://cks.nice.org.uk/urinary-tract-infection-lower-women#!topicsummary.

32. Milo G, Katchman EA, Paul M, *et al.* Duration of antibacterial treatment for uncomplicated urinary tract infection in women. *Cochrane Database Syst Rev* 2005; 2: CD004682.

33. Katchman EA, Milo G, Paul M, *et al.* Three-day vs. longer duration of antibiotic treatment for cystitis in women: systematic review and meta-analysis. *Am J Med* 2005; 118(11): 1196-207.

34. Barcella W, De Iorio M, Baio G, Malone-Lee JG. A Bayesian nonparametric model for white blood cells in patients with lower urinary tract symptoms. *Electron J Stat* 2016; 10(2): 3287-309.

35. Collins L, Sathiananthamoorthy S, Fader M, Malone-Lee J. Intermittent catheterisation after botulinum toxin injections: the time to reassess our practice. *Int Urogynecol J* 2017; 28(9): 1351-6.

36. Kass EH. Bacteriuria and pyelonephritis of pregnancy. *Arch Intern Med* 1960; 105: 194-8.

37. Savage WE, Hajj SN, Kass EH. Demographic and prognostic characteristics of bacteriuria in pregnancy. *Medicine (Baltimore)* 1967; 46(5): 385-407.

38. Kazemier BM, Koningstein FN, Schneeberger C, *et al.* Maternal and neonatal consequences of treated and untreated asymptomatic bacteriuria in pregnancy: a prospective cohort study with an embedded randomised controlled trial. *Lancet Infect Dis* 2015; 15(11): 1324-33.

39. Liou N, Currie J, James C, *et al.* Urothelial cells may indicate underlying bacteriuria in pregnancy at term: a comparative study. *BMC Pregnancy Childbirth* 2017; 17(1): 414.

40. Vogel JP, Lee AC, Souza JP. Maternal morbidity and preterm birth in 22 low- and middle-income countries: a secondary analysis of the WHO Global Survey dataset. *BMC Pregnancy Childbirth* 2014; 14: 56.

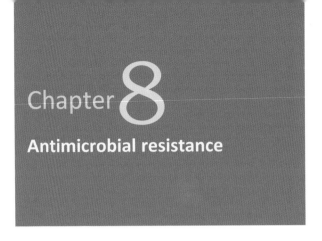

Chapter 8

Antimicrobial resistance

Charles Darwin and the story of the predictor moth (*Xanthopan morganii*)

We wish to introduce this chapter by discussing a remarkable story about Charles Darwin (Figure 8.1) because it is illustrative of a way of thinking that is important to how we approach the problem of AMR which is better grasped if explored with an eye to the mechanisms of evolution. There is another element; Darwin was a wonderful, careful conscientious scientist who sets us a compelling example of good practice. He wrote well and so his book *On the Origin of Species by Means of Natural Selection, or the Preservation of Favoured Races in the Struggle for Life*, published on 24 November 1859 [1], is not difficult; it makes an absorbing read.

One of the great stories about Charles Darwin is the predictor moth tale; a seminal lesson in the use of evidence, and how to think about and practice science. Despite being about an orchid and a moth it is most relevant to AMR. In any case, stories are a great way of learning about complicated facts and this tale is remarkable.

In 1861 Charles Darwin was on holiday with his family in Torquay. He became intrigued by the wild orchids growing near the shoreline. He began to study orchids in detail and through this developed ideas about the coevolution of orchids and the insects that pollinated them [2].

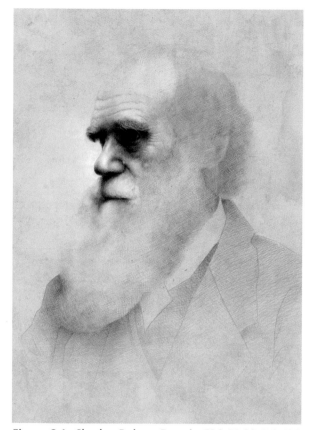

Figure 8.1. Charles Robert Darwin FRS FRGS FLS FZS (12 February 1809 - 19 April 1882). *On the Origin of Species by Means of Natural Selection, or the Preservation of Favoured Races in the Struggle for Life* was published on 24 November 1859. *Portrait by Alex Wilby.*

A friend, James Bateman from Madagascar, sent a specimen of *Angraecum sesquipedale* (Figure 8.2) in response to Darwin's requests made to acquaintances all over the world. *Angraecum sesquipedale* is also called Darwin's orchid, Christmas orchid, Star of Bethlehem orchid, and King of the Angraecums. Darwin noticed that the nectary was 12 inches long (Figure 8.2). The nectary is a tube that leads off the flower. It is far from full and the

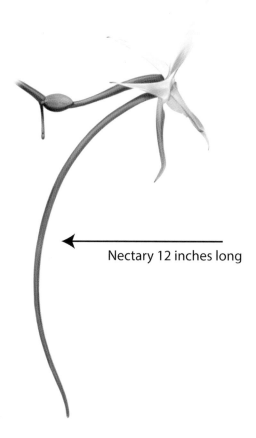

Nectary 12 inches long

Figure 8.2. *Angraecum sesquipedale*, **also known as Darwin's orchid, Christmas orchid, Star of Bethlehem orchid, and King of the Angraecums.** *Illustration courtesy of Alex Wilby.*

nectar occupies the lower 0.5cm. Thus, to access this, the moth must have a proboscis of sufficient length which it must insert up to the hilt. When it does so a release mechanism is activated and the flower deposits a sticky pollinia, onto the head parts of the insect. The pollen grains of the pollinia will be deposited on the anther of another flower that the moth subsequently visits. The mechanisms are exquisitely precise and highly evolved to ensure reliable pollination (Figure 8.3) [2].

Pollen grains in a waxy matrix

Delicate membrane
enclosing sticky pollinia
This is released onto the moth
head parts where it sticks

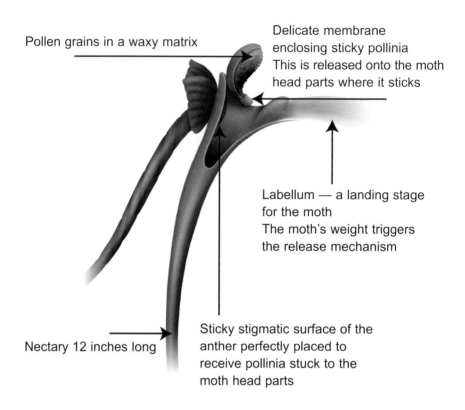

Labellum — a landing stage
for the moth
The moth's weight triggers
the release mechanism

Nectary 12 inches long

Sticky stigmatic surface of the
anther perfectly placed to
receive pollinia stuck to the
moth head parts

Figure 8.3. The parts of the orchid, *Angraecum sesquipedale*, as observed by Charles Darwin. *Illustration courtesy of Alex Wilby.*

Charles Darwin abducted a hypothesis of coevolution of species from his observations of orchid anatomy. Coevolution leads to specificity in flower and insect partnerships so as to focus the transporting of pollen within the floral species by providing the carrier insect with an exclusive source of nectar. From this hypothesis he deduced a famous prediction: in Madagascar, the home of *Angraecum sesquipedale*, there must live a moth with a proboscis of 12 inches in length that fed almost exclusively on the *Angraecum sesquipedale*.

Here is the crunch point: if this moth could be proved not to exist, the theory of evolution by natural selection would be refuted. In 1903, 16 years after Darwin had died, *Xanthopan morganii* (Morgan's sphinx moth) (Figure 8.4) was found with a 12-inch proboscis in Madagascar. It was named *Xanthopan morganii praedicta* in honour of this wager. In fact the "*praedicta*" suffix was a reference to Alfred Russell Wallace's suggestion

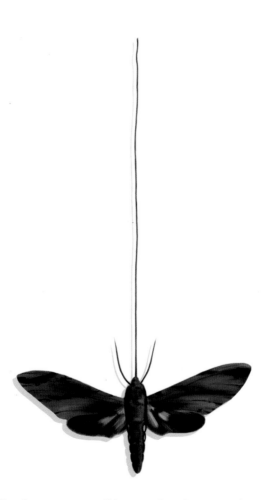

Figure 8.4. *Xanthopan morganii* (Morgan's sphinx moth), having a 12-inch proboscis, was found in Madagascar in 1903. *Illustration courtesy of Alex Wilby.*

that it would be a hawk moth. Thus, the two discoverers of evolution were remembered.

In 1992, thanks to the development of modern night-time methods, *Xanthopan morganii praedicta* was photographed feeding from *Angraecum sesquipedale* just as Darwin had predicted.

The "Orchid book" written by Charles Darwin and his son is a masterpiece of meticulous observational work that dissects out the extraordinary panoply of orchid sexual behaviour. The mechanisms are so beautifully described. It is a treatise on the astonishing power of evolution and a demonstration of the application of empirical science. Induction and abduction were carefully applied to formulate the hypothesis of coevolution amongst species. There followed the deduction of a prediction; the testing of this prediction was an exercise in falsification; refute the prediction and refute evolution (Figure 8.5). There is some beauty in the fact that the verification occurred after Darwin's death. Compare this tale to the hurried expediency, noisy bumptiousness and aggressive dogmatism of the conference circuits and you must wonder at the vandalisation of a crowning legacy.

The orchid came into being 112 million years ago, moths 130 million, mammals 200 million, and bacteria 3.5 billion years ago. There is plenty of time for mammals and bacteria to coevolve for mutual benefit. Humans and bacteria do coexist in commensal, symbiotic and mutualist relationships which may be vastly more complicated than we realise. The roots of trees function only because of the mutualist arrangement with the hyphae of fungi. *Escherichia coli* feeding in the human gut provide us with a supply of vitamin K; similarly, *Bacteroides thetaiotetraiotamicron* break down the complex polysaccharides in vegetables so that we can absorb the resulting monosaccharides. The bacteria in the normal bladder may play an important role in our health, the property invented by evolution but yet to be discovered by us. For 80 years we have slandered the bladder microbiome and nowadays, with the availability of molecular methods, we are in danger of doing the same to resistance genes through our premature extrapolations.

The *On the Origin of Species* and *On the Various Contrivances by which British and Foreign Orchids are Fertilised by Insects* books teach us the discipline of

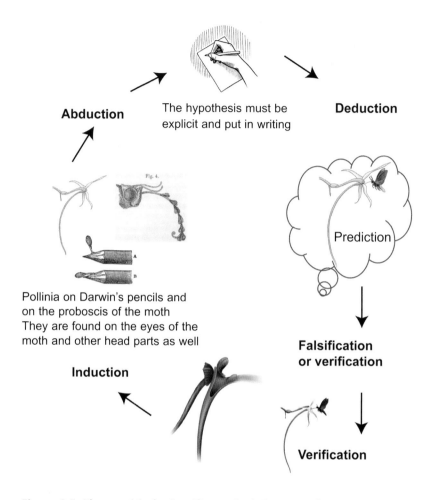

Abduction

The hypothesis must be explicit and put in writing

Deduction

Prediction

Pollinia on Darwin's pencils and on the proboscis of the moth They are found on the eyes of the moth and other head parts as well

Falsification or verification

Induction

Verification

Figure 8.5. The empirical scientific method that tested Darwin's theory of coevolution of the orchid and moth. This echoes the same *leitmotif* that has recurred several times through these pages. It is so important to our overall theme.

careful, reflective observation without hasty generalisations. There are no tests expedited out of between group differences, no regulations drawn up from crude extrapolations from inchoate observations. Everything is questioned, tested and re-examined to get to the truth. Consilience is used to examine the subject from different perspectives. You sense an enormous intellectual application, without ill-considered rush. It is well worth clinicians reading the *Origin of Species* book because it shows that there is so much more to science than a RCT, meta-analysis and p-values. Darwin was punished for his writing because it challenged dogmatic theological beliefs that were popular at that time. As always there were dissenters, but they struggled to be heard. Ironically, it was a Roman Catholic Augustinian friar and abbot who provided the material evidence for the mechanism of evolution — Father Gregor Johann Mendel (1822-1884).

We can bring these ideas into our subject: we think that the restrictive guidelines advocating 3-day treatment courses for uncomplicated UTI, with failures managed on culture, are mistaken and causing unnecessary chronic illness. It is an extravagant claim and should not rest as speculative extrapolation but be tested empirically. If we take our conjecture as a hypothesis, we may deduct a testable prediction conditioned on the hypothesis being true. So, we predict that there should be a detectable rise in the incidence of chronic cystitis, following the publication of guidelines, and commensurate with a change in prescribing practice. We tested this prediction and the results are described in Chapter 6, Figures 6.1 to 6.3, which demonstrate a marked rise in admissions for chronic cystitis, most notably interstitial cystitis when short course treatment for UTI was on the increase.

We have written on how patients with chronic recalcitrant bladder pain and recurrent cystitis can be diagnosed and treated, but at this time we have been unable to find a method that does not rely on the carefully monitored, extensive use of urinary antibiotics, given in full dose [3, 4]. As this book makes clear, we have used protracted courses of antibiotics, in some cases for several years, in order to manage the symptoms. We check efficacy, time and again, using trials without treatment. Once an effective regimen is found, response failure is rare. The commonest reason for prescription change is intolerance. We have never found cause to cycle antibiotics. We take on many patients said to suffer from alarming multi-resistant infections, but we treat them with first-generation, narrow-spectrum urinary antibiotics successfully, checking this by cessation trials. We are not complacent; despite the unreliability of the MSU culture we continue to arrange these to monitor resistance rates in the small number of isolates. Widely held opinions predict that we should be seeing much AMR and treatment failure, but this has not happened. Why should this be? These questions are not welcome. There is an accepted understanding of AMR and an intolerance of different perspectives. This does not serve a useful purpose; we must strive to improve our understanding by considering contradictory data.

Some do advocate that patients such as ours, for the common good, should not be treated for fear of a surge in AMR. Is it right to penalise a small subset of mainly women who suffer from an extremely unpleasant disease? An analysis of the facts about AMR may help to answer this.

Antimicrobial resistance

People with chronic UTI are not really the problem. Much greater difficulties are to be found in agricultural overuse in China, the USA, Brazil and the Asian subcontinent [5-7] — see ▦ Figure 8.6 [8].

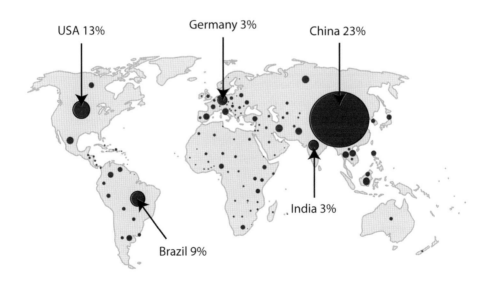

Figure 8.6. Antibiotic consumption for livestock production by country in 2013. The size of the icons are approximations. Van Boeckel *et al* [8].

In recent times it has been discovered that widespread multi-antibiotic resistance predates humans by millions of years [9-12]. This is not surprising; antibiotics are produced by microbes which use them to attack competitor species that are after the same sparse sources of nutrition. A microbe producing an antibiotic, must be resilient to its own aggression. Bacteria have been around for 3.5 billion years. Thus, the squabbling microbes have had ample time to coevolve ancient resistance factors to protect themselves and closely-related species from their particular weapons.

There is evidence for this: a section of the Lechuguilla Cave, New Mexico, has been sealed off from the rest of the world for 4 million years. Bacteria from this site are found resistant to many antibiotics; some multi-resistant to 14 currently prescribed agents [10]. Similar data have been obtained from deep bore holes into the Canadian permafrost [9] and deep ocean sampling [12]. What's more, Yanomami hunter-gatherers, isolated for 11,000 years, carry in their bowels microbes with numerous antimicrobial resistance genes including resistance to modern synthetic antibiotics [13]. These tribes are so isolated that they have had no medical antibiotic exposure, which reinforces the idea that such resistance is ancient and widely dispersed in the environment, pre-dating Alexander Fleming's discovery by millennia [14]. AMR is a Darwinian inevitability antedating humankind.

The current AMR crisis arises from the selection of resistant strains of the natural colonising populations. The selection pressure is created by antibiotic use and frequent misuse. The microbes in these mutualist, commensal or pathogenic populations can switch resistance genes on and off as needed in response to environmental stimulation. If bacteria manufacture resistance proteins, their nutritional demands rise commensurately, and they must pay an advantage cost. If they were to continue to express this resistance, once the offending antibiotic vacates the locality, the advantage cost would prove detrimental, the microbes disadvantaged, and their survival compromised. The influence of this effect is still being elucidated. To avoid this, they must switch off the relevant genes. On the other hand, if you maintain an environment with antibiotics, whether mixtures, broad- or narrow-spectrum agents, the microbes with relevant resistance genes will switch them on and thrive in those circumstances, despite the additional nutritional needs necessary to maintain this phenotype [15, 16]. This view is counter to two common misconceptions: 1) that treatment with antibiotics somehow "creates" new resistance; and 2) that the switching on of resistance is permanent [17].

Another misconception is that resistance data are a perfect reflection of what is occurring *in vivo*. If a patient consumes an antibiotic, the diagnostic cultures performed on their urine specimen will select ambient resistant bugs. This will happen, correspondingly with every antibiotic change. We now know from genomic studies, that cultures are not providing data on the causative organism, so the sensitivity tests may be irrelevant to disease treatment [18]. The normal bladder is not sterile, so a culture isolate may be innocent.

The normal bladder microbiome hosts over 500 different species, increasing by over approximately 10% in patients with cUTI [18]. UTI seems to be associated with an increase in species dispersion and an increase in microbial load but we know not what microbes are causing problems. Nevertheless, many are convinced that the microbes they isolate by culture or molecular methods are responsible for the infection. Because of this misunderstanding, the information about disease-related AMR available to us may be mistaken. These reports encourage clinicians to change an antibiotic prescription. This action will introduce a new selection pressure. The next culture will tell a different story, describing a different resistance set, the prescription is changed again and the selection pressure for greater resistance is built up. It cannot be said too often: a resistant microbe revealed by culture is the expected result of the selection pressure created by the antibiotic being taken, but it is not necessarily the cause of the disease. A consequence of this confusion is that a pessimistic view of UTI and the consequences of treatment gets promoted. The dependence on culture data results in patients being exposed to unnecessarily powerful regimens, which at worst are cycled.

In our tertiary referral clinic, we are dealing with some of the most complex chronic urinary tract infections in patients who have had considerable exposure to different antibiotics before they were referred here. Nevertheless, in 2014 we decided to stop treating on culture results. We had discovered the serious errors inherent in MSU culture [12], alongside clinical experience of unfavourable outcomes. From 2014, regardless of multi-resistance in the previous history, we stuck to first-generation, narrow-spectrum, urinary antibiotics, judging pathogen susceptibility on the clinical response and not culture [3, 4].

Measuring resistance

The considerations described are no reason not to be alert to AMR which is a most serious problem. We appreciated warnings from colleagues that we risked widespread resistance, and it worried us much. The exhortations gave us an hypothesis and a prediction to test: there should be a rising AMR trend amongst our patients.

Thus, we persisted in submitting urine samples for culture and watched the resistance data from the positive cultures. At our hospital, a significant culture involved the isolation of a pure growth of $\geq 10^5$ cfu/ml of a known urinary pathogen. Sensitivity tests were directed at those isolates and antibiotics that were tested routinely were amoxicillin, co-amoxiclav, ciprofloxacin, nitrofurantoin, and trimethoprim. For each positive culture we counted the occurrences of resistance to each of these antibiotics. There was thus a potential score range between zero antibiotics (no resistance) and all five antibiotics.

Between 2004 and 2018 we arranged 30,647 cultures of which 2547 (8%) grew $\geq 10^5$ cfu/ml of a single species of a known urinary pathogen. The very low isolation rate is well recognised in contemporary literature. These data were obtained from 3094 patients (mean age=61, sd=0.3). There were 2710 women and 384 men. For comparison purposes we collected data from patients attending the emergency department with symptoms of acute UTI between 2016 to 2018 providing 3648 positive cultures.

Figure 8.7 charts the mean number of antibiotics that were resisted, with 95% CI for the years 2004 to 2018.

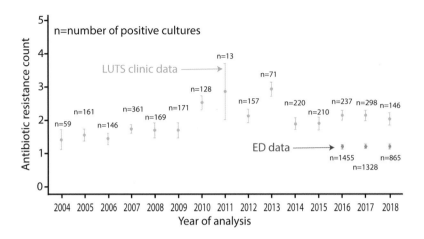

Figure 8.7. These plots of the mean number of antibiotics resisted, with 95% CI, provide data on annual returns. There are notable differences affecting some periods and they seem to reflect changes in clinic practice. We reported on 3094 LUTS clinic patients. We included 3648 patients who attended the emergency department with symptoms of an acute UTI so as to compare against the local community resistance rates. LUTS = Lower urinary tract symptoms clinic; ED = Emergency department.

The most striking difference affects the years 2010 to 2013 when we were focusing on the treatment of cUTI but treating on the results of sensitivity data obtained from the cultures. When we stopped using culture data the resistance counts fell significantly.

The legend of ▓ Figure 8.7 identifies the sample source: LUTS = Lower urinary tract symptoms clinic; ED = Emergency department. For the years 2004 to 2009 the LUTS clinic provided a traditional urodynamics and incontinence service with a growing interest in urinary tract infection which grew steadily through the decade. In 2010 we saw the start of an increase in referrals for cUTI in the wake of a series of publications from this centre [19, 20]. During 2010 to 2013 we used the results of sensitivity tests from routine MSU cultures and spun sediment cultures [21]. By January 2014 we became aware of data, now published [18], that cast great doubt on the validity of urine culture and its associated sensitivity tests. In response we excluded this from our practice, relying on symptoms and urine microscopy using a protocol based on simple, first-line urinary antibiotics [3]. There was a marked fall in our resistance rates (Kruskal-Wallis chi-squared = 164, df = 13, p-value <.001). In October 2015 the service was closed to new admissions [4], so that for 2016 to 2018 the data are enriched by patients receiving long-term care without new patients coming into the system. The lower resistance rates in the emergency department patients would reflect their limited exposure to antibiotics.

Figure 8.8 charts the results of positive MSU cultures from patients assessed over 10 visits to the service.

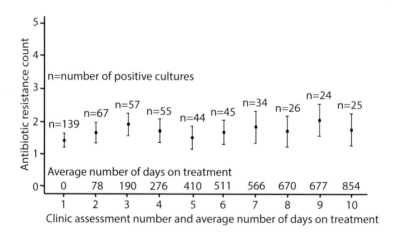

Figure 8.8. These plots of the mean number of antibiotics resisted are cross-sectional data obtained from a number of reviews in the clinics.

The more the visits, the longer the period of exposure to antibiotics. Thus, we are recording data after unusually protracted courses of treatment. There is a rise in resistance count at the first visit after starting antibiotics; this we should expect because of a selection effect from taking an antibiotic. There is no significant further rise after this occurrence; resistance is not increasing.

These data were obtained from a subset of 391 patients who presented new to the service after December 2013, when we ceased to use culture data. The sample size was smaller for three reasons:

- Because the service was closed to new admissions from October 2015 [4].
- Because only about 9% of our chronic patients test above the 10^5 cfu/ml threshold needed to trigger sensitivity testing.
- Only a minority of patients need such extensive follow-up (e.g. 854 days) so the numbers reduce with time.

Nevertheless, we collected sufficient data to power a meaningful analysis: the resistance at visit one differs from the other visits (Kruskal-Wallis chi-squared = 6.6701, df = 1, p-value 0.01). The key finding is that the resistance count rises marginally, with an effect size of 0.2 of an antibiotic, on starting treatment, and then remains on a plateau (1.7, 95% CI 1.6 to 1.8) throughout with no significant difference from visits 2 to 10. This phenomenon can be explained by a simple selection from a wild population that already carries resistance genes, such that once a patient is on an antibiotic, the cultures inevitably select out the resistant microbes. It is possible that the initial rise would be no different to that of an acute UTI sufferer receiving a one-off short-course treatment according to standard guidelines, but these studies have not been performed for comparison. What is clear is that longer-term treatment has no further exacerbating effect on AMR in urinary pathogens. Although we did not assess resistance rates in other niches such as the gut, skin and mouth, and acknowledge a possibility that such sites could harbour further AMR organisms, such matters do merit future scrutiny.

If our hypothesis that the antibiotic prescribed exerts a selection pressure on the results of a urine culture is correct, then we may predict a linear relationship between the amount of prescribing and a measure of resistance. If no such association exists, the hypothesis is refuted. There are many such data available in the literature. Figure 8.9 is a simplified abstraction of one example which we derived from Bronzwaer *et al* who reported a European surveillance project on blood culture data [22]. We have added a regression line with the dispersion of the estimate shaded. There is a correlation (R=0.6) as

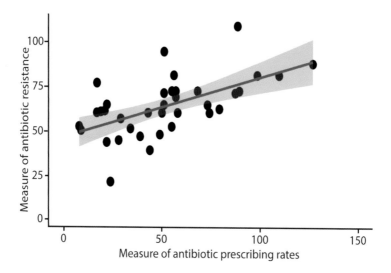

Figure 8.9. Antibiotic resistance measure as a function of prescriptions issued. Points represent different European countries. These data were abstracted from Bronzwaer et al [22].

If we hypothesise that antibiotic use causes cultures to select out microbes from the bladder microbiome that resist the antibiotic being consumed, then we should expect a correlation between antibiotic use and resistance rates as shown here. If this relationship were not found, the hypothesis would be refuted. We expect cultures to show isolates that resist the antibiotic being taken; we do not change the prescription.

occurs with the other similar examples. These correlations are frequently used to imply causation of AMR, which is wrong; there are other explanations. We proposed selection pressure from the treatment. The microbial resistance capacity may have existed for millennia and there is no saying that the isolate causes the disease.

The data presented in this chapter cast a different light on the matter of AMR. We have not seen the much-feared explosion in AMR arising from treating the patients of concern. There is evidence that treating on culture data may have encouraged more AMR and that contradicts the idea that precision of treatment, shaped by the sensitivities measured through culture, protects against AMR. That does not hold up anyway because the cultures do not address causation. The data reassure and do challenge those who believe that these patients should not be treated.

References

1. Darwin C. *On the origin of species by means of natural selection, or the preservation of favoured races in the struggle for life*. London: John Murray; 1859.

2. Darwin C. *On the various contrivances by which British and foreign orchids are fertilised by insects, and on the good effects of intercrossing*. London: John Murray; 1862: vi, 1, 365.

3. Swamy S, Barcella W, De Iorio M, *et al*. Recalcitrant chronic bladder pain and recurrent cystitis but negative urinalysis: what should we do? *Int Urogynecol J* 2018; 29(7): 1035-43.

4. Swamy S, Kupelian AS, Khasriya R, *et al*. Cross-over data supporting long-term antibiotic treatment in patients with painful lower urinary tract symptoms, pyuria and negative urinalysis. *Int Urogynecol J* 2019; 30(3): 409-14.

5. Klein EY, Van Boeckel TP, Martinez EM, *et al*. Global increase and geographic convergence in antibiotic consumption between 2000 and 2015. *Proc Natl Acad Sci USA* 2018; 115(15): E3463-70.

6. Van Boeckel TP, Brower C, Gilbert M, *et al*. Global trends in antimicrobial use in food animals. *Proc Natl Acad Sci USA* 2015; 112(18): 5649-54.

7. Van Boeckel TP, Gandra S, Ashok A, *et al*. Global antibiotic consumption 2000 to 2010: an analysis of national pharmaceutical sales data. *Lancet Infect Dis* 2014; 14(8): 742-50.

8. Van Boeckel TP, Glennon EE, Chen D, *et al*. Reducing antimicrobial use in food animals. *Science* 2017; 357(6358): 1350-2.

9. Perron GG, Whyte L, Turnbaugh PJ, *et al*. Functional characterization of bacteria isolated from ancient arctic soil exposes diverse resistance mechanisms to modern antibiotics. *PloS One* 2015; 10(3): e0069533.

10. Bhullar K, Waglechner N, Pawlowski A, *et al*. Antibiotic resistance is prevalent in an isolated cave microbiome. *PloS One* 2012; 7(4): e34953.

11. Brown MG, Balkwill DL. Antibiotic resistance in bacteria isolated from the deep terrestrial subsurface. *Microb Ecol* 2009; 57(3): 484-93.

12. Toth M, Smith C, Frase H, *et al*. An antibiotic-resistance enzyme from a deep-sea bacterium. *J Am Chem Soc* 2010; 132(2): 816-23.

13. Clemente JC, Pehrsson EC, Blaser MJ, *et al*. The microbiome of uncontacted Amerindians. *Sci Adv* 2015; 1(3): e1500183.

14. Hall BG, Barlow M. Evolution of the serine beta-lactamases: past, present and future. *Drug Resist Updat* 2004; 7(2): 111-23.

15. Wright GD. The antibiotic resistome: the nexus of chemical and genetic diversity. *Nat Rev Microbiol* 2007; 5(3): 175-86.

16. Blair JM, Webber MA, Baylay AJ, *et al*. Molecular mechanisms of antibiotic resistance. *Nat Rev Microbiol* 2015; 13(1): 42-51.

17. Ghosh D, Veeraraghavan B, Elangovan R, Vivekanandan P. Antibiotic resistance and epigenetics: more to it than meets the eye. *Antimicrob Agents Chemother* 2020; 64(2): e02225-19.

18. Sathiananthamoorthy S, Malone-Lee J, Gill K, *et al*. Reassessment of routine midstream culture in diagnosis of urinary tract infection. *J Clin Microbiol* 2019; 57(3): 01452-18.

19. Khasriya R, Khan S, Lunawat R, *et al*. The inadequacy of urinary dipstick and microscopy as surrogate markers of urinary tract infection in urological outpatients with lower urinary tract symptoms without acute frequency and dysuria. *J Urol* 2010; 183(5): 1843-7.

20. Kupelian AS, Horsley H, Khasriya R, *et al*. Discrediting microscopic pyuria and leucocyte esterase as diagnostic surrogates for infection in patients with lower urinary tract symptoms: results from a clinical and laboratory evaluation. *BJU Int* 2013; 112(2): 231-8.

21. Khasriya R, Sathiananthamoorthy S, Ismail S, *et al*. Spectrum of bacterial colonization associated with urothelial cells from patients with chronic lower urinary tract symptoms. *J Clin Microbiol* 2013; 51(7): 2054-62.

22. Bronzwaer SL, Cars O, Buchholz U, *et al*. A European study on the relationship between antimicrobial use and antimicrobial resistance. *Emerg Infect Dis* 2002; 8(3): 278-82.

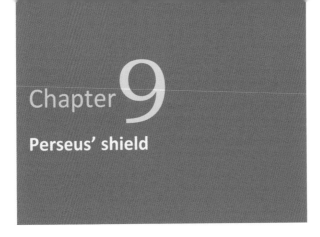

Chapter 9

Perseus' shield

The title of this chapter was used for our first conference abstract on the epithelial cells found in the urine. As a basic science paper, we were allocated the graveyard slot at the end of the conference. We call it the "kissy session" because the audience consists only of the presenting teams, and as each finishes they trawl sparse rows kissing their colleagues goodbye, thus heading for home. The last paper tends to be presented to the chairmen, janitor, and your research team. Always remember to kiss the janitors; it is greatly appreciated.

Medusa was one of three monstrous Gorgons who were winged creatures with living venomous serpents for their hair. If you gazed into Medusa's eyes you were turned into stone, so that there was little chance of you changing your mind after that. Polydectes had fallen in love with Perseus' mother, but Perseus did not approve of this match so Polydectes thought to remove Perseus by trapping him into taking on Medusa. In the event, Perseus got around the problem by using Medusa's reflection in his polished shield to guide him whilst he decapitated her safely. You might be interested to know that Pegasus and a golden sword came out of Medusa's neck; whilst admittedly a bit odd, it did provide Perseus with some transport and some quality, military hardware. Our metaphor arises because of our suspicion that the shield-like urinary urothelial cells (Figure 9.1) may reflect the pathology of chronic UTI.

There are worries about contamination of a urine sample by bacteria from the vagina and perineal skin. For a long time, it has been assumed that if epithelial cells are seen in the urine sample, they imply skin contamination

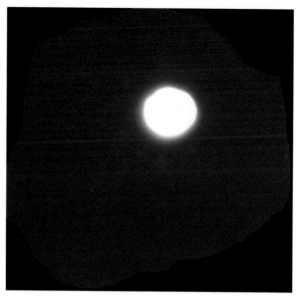

Figure 9.1. An electron micrograph demonstrating a uroepithelial cell stained by DAPI which is taken up by DNA, hence the glowing nucleus. The cell has scalloped edges with Anglo-Saxon shield-like qualities, trendy at the battle of Edlington (AD 878), albeit a little late for Perseus. *Micrograph courtesy of Harry Horsley.*

and the sample is thus rejected. Much effort is expended in trying to achieve samples that are free of epithelial cells and studies that use these as outcome measures have settled for catheter specimens of urine (CSU) as the superior option over the MSU or a simple pee into a pot [1]. Study of the literature reveals an interesting fact; the accuracy of epithelial cells in identifying contamination was never validated. Until recently it was simply a surmise free from evidence.

There is a way of exploring this. Uroplakins (UPs) are a group of transmembrane proteins that are found in the cells of the urothelium and nowhere else. Therefore, uroplakin-III (UP3), which we can label using an immunofluorescence technique, acts to mark a cell as originating from the lining of the urinary tract and not the skin. Figure 9.2 is a micrograph of a

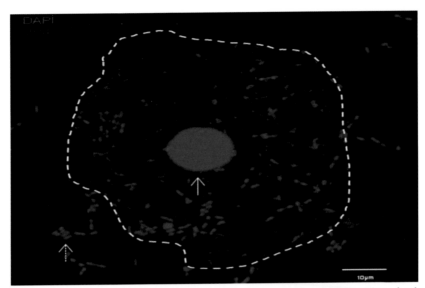

Figure 9.2. This is a laser scanning confocal image of a UP3-positive shed urothelial cell. The red is the UP3 and the blue is the DNA stained by DAPI; some microbes are showing up as well. The solid arrow points to the nucleus and the dashed arrow, bacteria. Without the correct staining, folds in the cell membrane can be confused with bacteria.

In the studies that we have conducted on urinalysis, the proportion of UP3-positive cells of the epithelial cells counted ranged from 0.7 to 0.9. This belies the view that these cells are markers of contamination. But that is not all; these cells tell us a great deal about our specimen collection techniques. Micrograph courtesy of Harry Horsley.

cell that we obtained from a person's urine stained in this way and then examined by laser scanning confocal microscopy. We have used this method to analyse the epithelial cells identified in the urine of our patients. To our astonishment, we have found that over 90% [1, 2] of these cells are UP3 positive which puts pay to the assumption that these are skin cells and indicative of contamination. That is a big mistake and we shall learn that they are certainly not markers of contamination.

Hyperplasia is an increase in the number of epithelial cells as a result of cell proliferation. This is a ubiquitous physiological response of epithelia to stress

219

and chronic inflammation is a common cause. This is illustrated in ▨ Figure 6.13. If in this process, the cells change their form as with urothelial cells changing to keratinised squamous cells, then this is called metaplasia.

We are seeing evidence of chronic inflammation of the urothelium and urethra, and so we should expect to see signs of hyperplasia affecting these tissues. It is evident in animal models of cystitis [3] which show that bacterial cystitis is associated with hyperplasia, apoptosis and exfoliation of urothelial cells [4]. Thus, we tested the hypothesis that our patients should demonstrate an increased number of urothelial cells in the urine.

▨ Figure 9.3 is a plot of the data obtained from those experiments [5]. We studied normal controls and patients with LUTS with or without pyuria. There

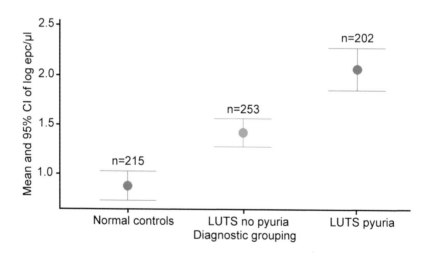

Figure 9.3. The mean log epithelial cell counts and 95% CI levels from controls and LUTS patients with and without pyuria.

It appears that instead of being contaminants these cells are significant markers of the disease. There is an increase in epithelial cell shedding in patients with symptoms of cUTI whether or not they have pyuria.

220

is an obvious difference between these groups manifesting increased cell shedding associated with disease.

In Chapter 6 we described the pathology of bacterial parasitisation of urothelial cells which was originally described in mice. In humans, we have demonstrated microbes parasitising these cells as part of the pathology of bacterial cystitis [5].

Figure 9.4 shows a clue cell which is a urothelial cell with bacteria attached to or inside the cell. Figure 9.5 is a monochrome confocal

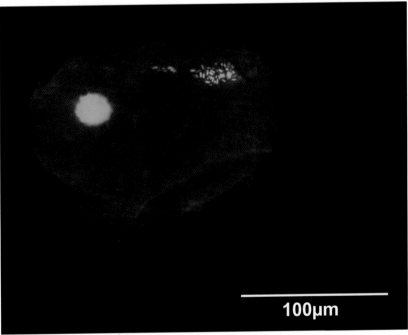

Figure 9.4. A confocal micrograph demonstrating a urothelial cell; the DAPI stain is taken up by DNA so that the nucleus and bacteria fluoresce. This is a two-dimensional image so we may not say whether the bacteria are adherent to the urothelial cell or whether they colonise the interior. Confocal microscopic studies show that they do both [5]. The colour of the immunofluorescence is dictated by the choice of lasers and filters. *Micrograph courtesy of Harry Horsley.*

Nuclear DNA stained by DAPI immunofluorescence under laser illumination with confocal microscopy

Bacterial DNA stained by DAPI showing up through immunofluorescence

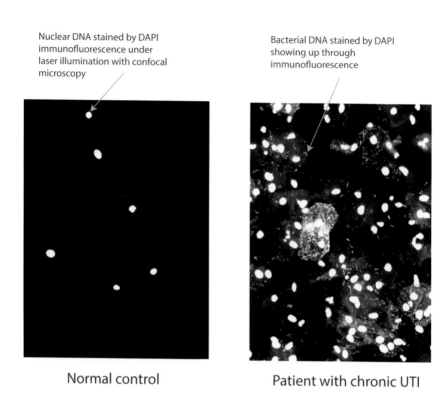

Normal control   Patient with chronic UTI

Figure 9.5. A confocal micrograph of DAPI stained urothelial cells from a normal control and from a patient with cUTI.

These are human urothelial cells from a urinary spun sediment preparation. The microscopy is done by confocal imaging and a fluorescent staining protocol uses DAPI to expose the DNA. The control cells therefore only reveal their nuclei. With the patient we can see bacteria associated with the cells and there are many more cells evident. These are clue cells. We cannot tell whether the microbes adhere to the surface or are inside their host cell. We should not assume that these microbes are necessarily causing the cUTI; they may be fulfilling an entirely innocent role. Micrographs courtesy of Harry Horsley.

micrograph of DAPI stained cells from a normal control and from a patient with cUTI. DAPI (4′,6-diamidino-2-phenylindole) is a fluorescent DNA stain that is excited by 405nm laser light which we can apply using the confocal

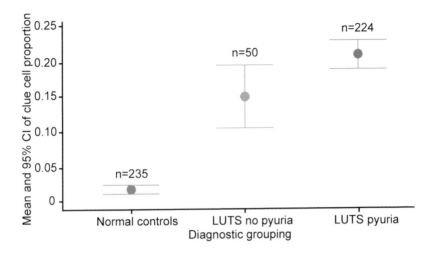

Figure 9.6. The mean and 95% CI levels of the proportion of clue cells in LUTS patients with and without pyuria compared with controls.

For this analysis we counted all of the uroepithelial cells per µl of urine and then counted the clue cells identified by DAPI staining and calculated the proportion of uroepithelial cells that were clue cells. As we have shown that the number of epithelial cells is elevated in the patient groups, so is the proportion parasitised by bacteria.

microscope. Because the stain is only taken up by DNA, nuclear and bacterial, the cell nuclei fluoresce as do bacteria. We studied the proportion of clue cells expressed in counts from patients and controls [6]. Figure 9.6 illustrates the results of that analysis.

The image shown in Figure 9.4 must be viewed with caution. It is two-dimensional so we do not know whether the bacteria are inside or outside of the cell. We need to deploy a technique that can resolve that for us. In the past we used an antibiotic protection assay whereby we kill off all extracellular microbes, with an exclusively extracellular antibiotic such as gentamicin. We then wash the preparation, lyse the cells and perform cultures on the lysate. Thus, we first demonstrated evidence of intracellular bacterial colonisation of human urothelial cells [7]. Coincidentally, the data showed why intravesical gentamicin might be ill-advised.

A more direct method is to use confocal microscopy. The illumination for a confocal laser scanning microscope comes from lasers which excite fluorescent dyes and proteins. The microscopist decides what regions of the specimen should be explored and only those are exposed to the laser illumination. The microscope is able to scrutinise sections through the depths of a specimen, layer by layer without interference with those parts not in focus. This differential depth resolution operates along a z-axis (top/bottom) complementing the x-axis (left/right) and the y-axis (up/down). A computer stores the images forming a z-stack and this can be manipulated to achieve a three-dimensional image of the specimen. This enables us to see where microbes that have parasitised cells are located (Figure 9.7). The confocal microscopy is supported by a computer and that enables us to build 3D block images of the cell or tissue under observation. Thus, Figure 9.8 is a construct from the human urothelial organoid [8] that we use in our laboratories to study the interaction of the urothelium with microbes and the chemistry of the environment. This image shows bacterial colonies forming inside of the urothelial cells.

Let us now link these sophisticated images with what happens in our clinic. We use an ordinary school laboratory light microscope, an Olympus CX23, and a Neubauer haemocytometer counting chamber. There is no staining or centrifuging but we conduct the examination in the clinic because white blood cells lyse soon after collection. What we see is illustrated in Figure 9.9. The return of traditional microscopy to clinical areas would be a tall order so we have been working on adapting artificial intelligence (AI) to robotic microscopy. Amazingly, AI is teaching us that the urinary cellular sediment is a much richer source of valuable data than we imagined. We do hope that robotics will reintroduce urine microscopy into much wider acceptance.

So, we have a situation where patients with LUTS and pyuria, suspected of suffering from chronic UTI, who when compared with controls are shown to be exfoliating increased numbers of uroepithelial cells. We know that they are urothelial cells because over 90% stain positive to uroplakin-III (UP3) [1, 2].

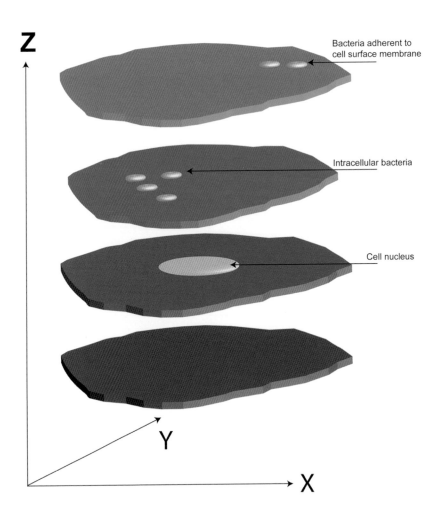

Z

Bacteria adherent to
cell surface membrane

Intracellular bacteria

Cell nucleus

Y

X

Figure 9.7. A confocal microscopic z-stack image of a uroepithelial cell which enables us to observe different planes through the thickness of the cell. Differential immunofluorescent staining enhances the information that can be obtained. In this example we depict a z-stack with the nucleus showing in the centre of the cell and clusters of bacteria on the cell surface and deeper inside. *Illustration by James Malone-Lee.*

Harry Horsley's human urothelial organoid
for laboratory studies of living tissue *in vitro*

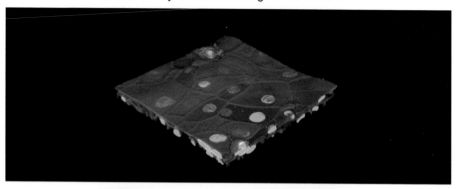

These are all confocal micrographic images

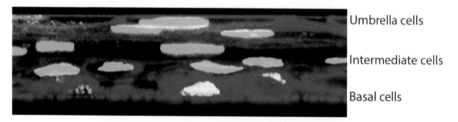

Umbrella cells

Intermediate cells

Basal cells

Intracellular
bacterial colony
next to nucleus

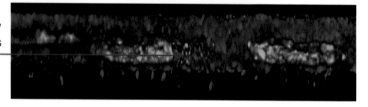

Figure 9.8. Confocal micrographic images obtained from our human urothelial organoid demonstrating bacterial colonies inside the urothelial cells. *Micrographs courtesy of Harry Horsley.*

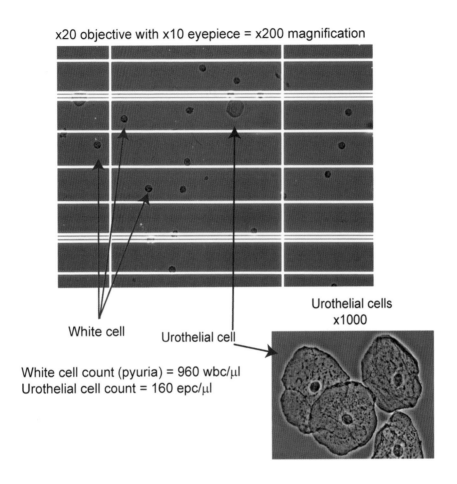

x20 objective with x10 eyepiece = x200 magnification

Urothelial cells
x1000

White cell   Urothelial cell

White cell count (pyuria) = 960 wbc/μl
Urothelial cell count = 160 epc/μl

Figure 9.9. Clinic microscopy (using an Olympus CX23) of a fresh, unspun, unstained specimen of urine in a Neubauer haemocytometer. This is what we see. This method was used to collect the data illustrated in Figure 9.3.

By labelling the cell membrane and using the simple DNA counterstain, DAPI, confocal microscopy shows a proportion of these cells to have bacteria colonising their surface and/or interior. We called these "clue cells" because they were so reminiscent of a similar phenomenon seen in vaginal cells typically when bacterial vaginosis is caused by *Gardnerella vaginalis*. In our case by contrast they are bladder cells. There is a greater proportion of these found in cUTI patients compared with controls. We have shown that cultures of concentrates of these cells show increased bacterial loads in the patients [7]. We have also found that during the course of a normal pregnancy there is a notable increase in cell exfoliation [2]. The hyperplasia of the urothelium which feeds this exfoliation causes us to pose two questions that are burning to be answered. Is the ultrasound finding of bladder wall thickness a manifestation of infection-associated hyperplasia of the urothelium [9]? What is the morphology of the cells that make up the trigonal metaplasia seen on cystoscopy?

The discovery that the urinary epithelial cells were not indicators of specimen contamination, but important markers of bacterial cystitis, caused us to mourn the numerous MSU specimens condemned to rejection by laboratories all over the world; what savagery. It also motivated us to examine the whole process of sample collection and to re-evaluate the assumptions about contamination [1].

Figure 9.10 is an illustration of a bladder that is affected by an inflammatory state. The reaction results in an accumulation, under gravity, at the bladder neck of a deposit of the exfoliated cells, white blood cells and debris resulting from this immune response. This sediment must offer nutrition for saprophytic commensals living in the microbiome and so we should expect this to trigger an increase in the numbers of urinary planktonic microbes. That is a hypothesis yet to be tested.

Since the deposit is created by the disease process and we know that it contains parasitised urothelial cells it might be thought that this concentrate would make an excellent substrate for identifying the aetiology of the infection. The problem is that it is passed out in the first part of the stream which is rejected in favour of collecting a midstream specimen of urine. Figures 9.11 to 9.14 take us through the voiding process in order to illustrate this phenomenon. The images are taken from our published work on this matter [1].

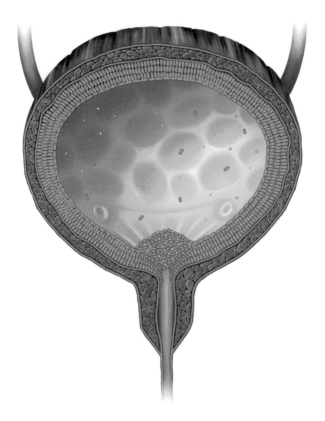

Figure 9.10. The bladder with an inflammatory sediment collecting at the base.

The innate immune response causes an inflammatory exudate of exfoliated urothelial cells, white and red blood cells, along with various proteins, lipids and sugars to accumulate at the bladder neck because of gravity. This sediment will provide a feeding substrate to many saprophytes that are likely to thrive on this bounty. This may in turn influence the results of a quantitative urine culture but the abundant microbes may not be the cause of the infection, but a consequence. However, it is no less probable that the parasitising culprits are contained in the shed cells. Illustration courtesy of Alex Wilby.

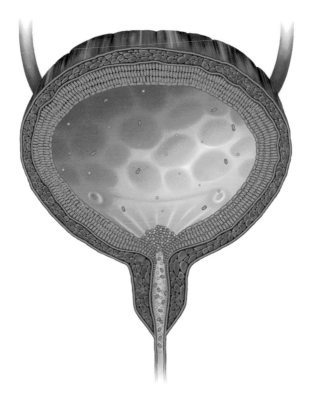

Figure 9.11. The bladder and the first void.

The first part of the void which contains the richest source of pathological information is passed out first. Unfortunately, this is discarded when a midstream specimen of urine is collected on the assumption that it is contaminated. The evidence [1] implies that it is not so contaminated and has the potential to tell us much about the disease of interest. Illustration courtesy of Alex Wilby.

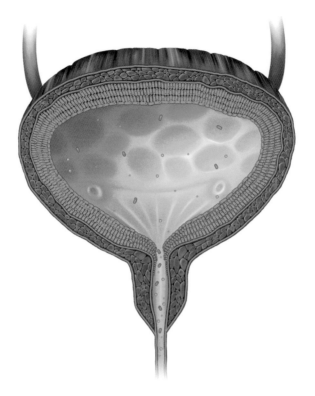

Figure 9.12. The midstream urine specimen of the bladder.

The midstream specimen is deficient in the inflammatory sediment and the exfoliated and parasitised urothelial cells that ought to be the focus of disease exploration. Our well-intentioned protocols for ensuring a sample that is least contaminated cause us to miss most of the footprints left behind by the pathology. Illustration courtesy of Alex Wilby.

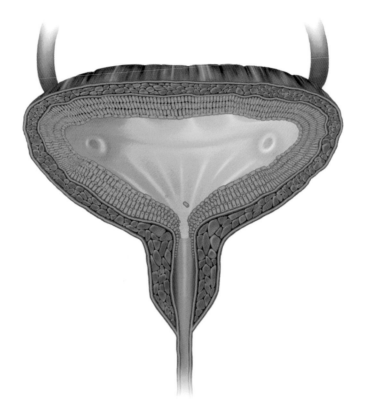

Figure 9.13. The terminal stream.

By now the sample, which is significantly clarified, makes for a fair approximation to a catheter specimen of urine (CSU). In the next image we consider the implications for the CSU. Illustration courtesy of Alex Wilby.

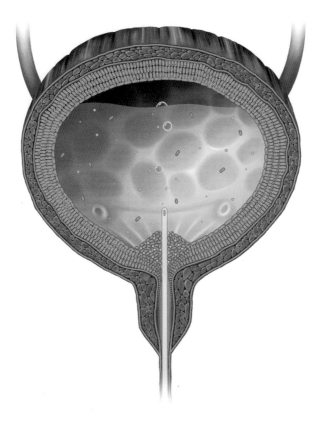

Figure 9.14. The catheter specimen of urine.

This image shows how the catheter passes through the pathological concentrate at the bladder base and rises above it to sample a substrate diluted by the urine and cleansed by gravity. We have done the science on this and found that this is exactly what happens. Illustration courtesy of Alex Wilby.

If you stain the cells of the spun sediment taken from a urine sample you can show the UP3-positive cells, count them along with other epithelial cells and express the cells of urothelial origin as a proportion of all the cells. This calculation of the proportion of UP3 cells is the crucial measure. The more contamination that there is, the lower this proportion must be. We were shocked to find that in comparing an ordinary void, with a midstream specimen and a catheter sample, this contamination measure did not differ. The catheter specimens achieved the sparsest of culture results. The greatest return on bacterial isolation was achieved from a simple straight void into a collecting bowl. The clinical significance of the isolates must wait on someone solving the causation problem. What we can say is that the assumptions that resulted in the widely adopted specimen collection guidelines were wrong [1].

What does all this mean?

The important question is: does any of this matter? It is a pleasure to answer that because we do not yet know! We are not going to extemporise answers created from plausible explanations. There is much empirical science to do before we can address the many of the questions that arise from these discoveries. We have shown that the cells are not contaminants; they bear pathological messages, and the assumptions about specimen collection, which will influence how we may harvest them, have been refuted. There is something else which is illustrated in a rather typical record obtained from one of our patients (Figure 9.15). The epithelial cell counts correlate with the pyuria; the plots are not always so in phase, but the counts tend to vary in a similar pattern during the response to the treatment of disease. These cells are easy to harvest so they offer a wonderful opportunity for much future clinic research.

We should rather take hemlock than suggest that counting these cells be promoted as some kind of diagnostic test. We all need a long sojourn, free from the horrors of another diagnostic test proposal.

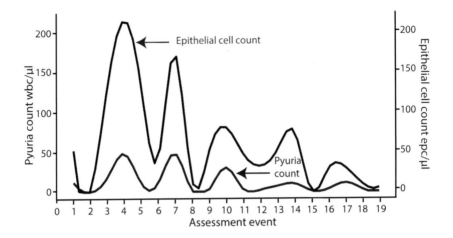

Figure 9.15. A plot of the pyuria and epithelial cell counts recorded from a patient under treatment for a chronic UTI. The epithelial cell counts (red) and pyuria (blue) are correlated but a little out of phase. The oscillations in the counts are well shown and they tend to settle similarly as the disease continues to come under control. This is a most typical example and emphasises the fact that these cells are not contaminants but important indicators of the disease activity.

References

1. Collins L, Sathiananthamoorthy S, Rohn J, Malone-Lee J. A revalidation and critique of assumptions about urinary sample collection methods, specimen quality and contamination. *Int Urogynecol J* 2020; 31(6): 1255-62.

2. Liou N, Currie J, James C, *et al.* Urothelial cells may indicate underlying bacteriuria in pregnancy at term: a comparative study. *BMC Pregnancy Childbirth* 2017; 17(1): 414.

3. Uchida K, Samma S, Rinsho K, *et al.* Stimulation of epithelial hyperplasia in rat urinary bladder by *Escherichia coli* cystitis. *J Urol* 1989; 142(4): 1122-6.

4. Thumbikat P, Berry RE, Zhou G, *et al.* Bacteria-induced uroplakin signaling mediates bladder response to infection. *PLoS Pathog* 2009; 5(5): e1000415.

5. Horsley H, Malone-Lee J, Holland D, *et al*. *Enterococcus faecalis* subverts and invades the host urothelium in patients with chronic urinary tract infection. *PloS One* 2013; 8(12): e83637.

6. Gill K, Kang R, Sathiananthamoorthy S, *et al*. A blinded observational cohort study of the microbiological ecology associated with pyuria and overactive bladder symptoms. *Int Urogynecol J* 2018; 29(10): 1493-500.

7. Khasriya R, Sathiananthamoorthy S, Ismail S, *et al*. Spectrum of bacterial colonization associated with urothelial cells from patients with chronic lower urinary tract symptoms. *J Clin Microbiol* 2013; 51(7): 2054-62.

8. Horsley H, Dharmasena D, Malone-Lee J, Rohn JL. A urine-dependent human urothelial organoid offers a potential alternative to rodent models of infection. *Sci Rep* 2018; 8(1): 1238.

9. Tafuro L, Montaldo P, Iervolino LR, *et al*. Ultrasonographic bladder measurements can replace urodynamic study for the diagnosis of non-monosymptomatic nocturnal enuresis. *BJU Int* 2010; 105(1): 108-11.

Chapter 10

Children

We ought to include a chapter on children in a book on cystitis but we have to approach this in constrained circumstances. Our service and the associated scientific programme grew out of an incontinence service founded in 1981. We had treated children for 35 years, dealing with diurnal incontinence and nocturnal enuresis. The practice grew out of the fact that clinicians were unattracted to the subject and there was a paucity of treatment centres; we filled the gap. As we found in adults, we identified problems with the exclusion of the UTI diagnosis using conventional methods. We were accepting referrals of children with similar histories to the adult patients and we were managing them through similar approaches to treatment. Our caseload was small, and with the long history of the centre our caring for children seemed unremarkable. The fact appeared on our service returns and our staff attended appropriate training.

In October 2015 our clinic was closed down for 6 weeks, this being a skirmish in the long-running dipstick wars [1]. We reopened in response to a High Court order following an action brought by our patients.

On the day of the court case we received the following instruction by NHS seniors:

"In every case in which you are treating a child, or advising on the treatment of a child, the clinical management, and any significant change in the clinical management, has been [sic] discussed with and agreed with a named consultant paediatrician before it is put into practice. That discussion and agreement should be contemporaneously and retrievably documented in the clinical notes."

This was welcome to us because we had long craved involvement of a paediatrician in our service and thought the stipulation might encourage this. In the event, we failed to find a paediatrician willing to do so. Our superiors proposed a consultant, working in another part of the country, who advised that we return to dipsticks and culture which contradicted our science. Another advised that we send all our extant paediatric patients back to the GP. The tempestuous reaction of GPs to the recent clinic closure showed that option to be unviable. A kind and generous paediatrician agreed to review our treatment but limited comment to acknowledging the receipt of our reports. With that good person's help, we were able to complete treatment of extant patients and reduce our paediatric caseload to zero. It was evident that our local commissioners aspired to this outcome. We are able to reassure you, reader, that all of our case notes on quondam child patients were reviewed with a fine tooth-comb: we were not found to have transgressed.

We have been contacted by parents who believe their children to be suffering similarly to the adults described in this book. We have not seen nor diagnosed those children. We must own up to causing dismay by declining involvement in the campaigns and actions organised by those parents. Where we have commented we have referred enquirers to the peer-reviewed published literature. The literature reports that paediatricians have identified similar problems with diagnosis to those that affect the adults [2].

We have been made all too aware of the strength of feelings on this matter. It would therefore be wrong for us to discuss the pathophysiology and treatment of UTI in children. Instead, we shall discuss the comments that have been made by others, with better credentials than us, who have been co-opted into this debate.

First, we paraphrase the comments made by a senior paediatrician at a meeting for parents and managers where the implications of the restriction on our service was being discussed:

> We understand your frustration; you are parents advocating for your child and you are only doing your best. However, we consultants will vary in our approaches. Where a child is concerned we would always want the involvement of a paediatrician because children are not like adults and their pathology is different. We paediatricians have fought for this and the Royal College of Paediatrics and Child Health would recommend a paediatrician be co-opted when another specialist is treating a child.

> We are not opposed to new ideas, innovations and new thinking but there are government structures that control all this and there are restrictions and rules that ensure that we do not start treatments without regulation of some sort. We have to check that things are being done the right way, otherwise in ten years' time we might regret what we are doing.

> We have an epi-urological approach to your children so we would expect to do a urine dipstick and urine culture, and microscopy might well play a role. We are used to seeing patients like your children who have been through a whole host of organisations, specialists and investigations. We may have to think outside the box, adopting a holistic approach looking at the complete story realising that it is not just one diagnosis.

A senior director, also a paediatrician, spent time with worried parents and put effort into exploring the options available. Here we paraphrase the response that the parents received:

> We understand your feelings and worries as parents of children with these chronic symptoms. We all agree that good practice requires the assessment of children by a multidisciplinary team

offering a holistic approach to treatment informed by NICE guidelines, pathways and international evidence. We would expect involvement of local paediatricians and the mental health services. A child should be assessed first before being treated. Parents should consult their GP about referral to secondary and tertiary paediatric services and there is the NHS Choice Framework.

The Royal College of Paediatrics and Child Health (RCPCH) responded to enquiries from concerned parents with a letter which we paraphrase:

The writer explained the role of the College and then went on to emphasise the importance of NICE guidelines and expert panels working with evidence. The letter described a need for periodic multidisciplinary paediatric assessment that included specialists in mental and emotional health, the GP and schools. This would ensure an accurate diagnosis provided that all the clinical data were available. The writer said that since the problem was a rare condition, there was a case for more research into this condition.

So why these comments? What on earth caused such important people and their organisations to become involved in this arena? We have been told many times that whether in adults or children, our speciality is most unappealing to our colleagues. It is far from prestigious. Worldwide academic clinicians committing to this fulltime are numbered less than the fingers of a hand. So how could our pathetic little dipstick war erupt into the High Court [3], the national press [4], the House of Commons of the UK Parliament [5] and so much more? Whilst our superiors suspected us of subversive scheming it is particularly relevant that we were never part of the agitation; academics should stick to the science. Thus, to us, these extraordinary events look like a reflection of "New Power" [6]; a social shift, transforming our culture and battering the old hierarchies. Heimans and Timms' book *New Power: Why Outsiders are Winning, Institutions are Failing, and How the Rest of Us Can Keep Up in the Age of Mass Participation* is worth a read. Facebook, Twitter and similar media are supporting networks of people with common interest. Patients and parents can share experiences, research, sift opinions and build alliances equipped to challenge "Old Power". Whilst it might have been so in the past, we do not believe that the problems of UTI in children will close with the statements above. Our doubts originate from our experience of "New Power" which pressured us into thinking differently about our management methods for adults and those influences we continue to experience every day. A telling prompt are witness narratives such as that reproduced below. Nowadays, these stories are widely available on social media sites and one route of access is through the patients' organisations described in Chapter 7.

We were keen to allow a patient to contribute her story to this chapter but given the circumstances felt that it would be disingenuous to reproduce one such written by a child. Thus, below, we reproduce the text of a letter that one of our young adult patients wrote for the Royal College of Paediatrics and Child Health. Her symptoms record is reproduced in ▨ Figure 7.6.

A young adult writes of her experiences as a child:

"I developed a chronic UTI as a result of recurrent childhood urinary infections which were repeatedly misdiagnosed and left untreated, resulting in severe bladder and kidney symptoms which left me with a misdiagnosis of interstitial cystitis. I am now 22 years old and this condition has stripped me of my entire childhood.

"I started to develop symptoms of severe urinary frequency and urgency when I was 6 years old. When my parents initially took me to see my GP, a urine dipstick was carried out and showed no signs of infection. A subsequent culture showed insignificant bacterial growth, resulting in no further treatment. When my symptoms subsequently worsened over the next 3 months, further negative dipsticks and cultures were carried out and I was misdiagnosed with overactive bladder syndrome. By this time, my urinary frequency had progressed to the point where I was urinating every 10 minutes and could not be away from a toilet for any length of time. My parents and school teachers were advised to encourage me to train my bladder to hold more urine by withholding access to a toilet, which resulted in such severe pain and embarrassment that I became terrified of going to school and missed a significant amount of my primary school education.

"Coincidentally, recurrent ear infections throughout my childhood meant that I was prescribed numerous short courses of antibiotics, which somewhat helped to reduce my bladder symptoms. However, my symptoms would recur quickly after the antibiotic course was finished. Despite this clear correlation in symptoms, any suggestion of an infection was dismissed repeatedly by my GP.

"I battled through my teenage years with fluctuating bladder symptoms that often left me leaving the classroom several times during school lessons and avoiding school trips and social interaction for fear of suffering bladder symptoms. When I was 17, I suddenly developed a severe worsening of symptoms, resulting in immense burning during urination, severe urgency, severe bladder pain and a sensation that I had a boiling hot marble stuck in my urethra. I saw my GP, who diagnosed me with a UTI based on my symptoms and prescribed me with a week-long course of antibiotics. However, despite a slight improvement in my symptoms during this time, the symptoms continued to linger. When my GP subsequently sent my urine off for culture, it revealed mixed growth of doubtful significance, and I was diagnosed with "post-UTI irritation" and placed on oxybutynin. This pattern of events continued to repeat over the next 3 months, with numerous short 3-day courses of antibiotics, oxybutynin, Vesicare and amitriptyline being prescribed in an attempt to relieve my pain.

"Over the course of the next 2 years, my symptoms continued to worsen. I saw my GP hundreds of times and was referred to a total of two urogynaecologists and two urologists, all of whom either diagnosed me with overactive bladder or interstitial cystitis, and one of whom claimed that my symptoms were psychological in nature and that my brain was simply "wired differently" to everyone else. I underwent two urodynamic studies, three KUB ultrasounds and two rigid cystoscopies under anaethestic, the second of which I also underwent a ureteroscopy, retrograde study, urethral dilation, ureter dilation and bladder distension following a misdiagnosis of kidney stones after a poor-quality CT scan. Unfortunately, these investigations caused a massive deterioration in my symptoms and I was hospitalised on multiple occasions with severe uncontrollable pain and vomiting, kidney infections, urinary retention and passing frank blood clots that were so thick that I was unable to pass urine. Each time I was admitted to hospital and given IV antibiotics, my symptoms would improve dramatically, only to relapse as soon as the course had finished.

"By the time I self-referred myself to ***** private clinic in 2015, I was near suicidal with pain. My symptoms included severe, debilitating pain in my urethra, bladder, kidneys and vagina, urine retention that frequently left me unable to pass urine for 24 hours at a time, significant voiding issues and incredible urgency which felt as though my bladder was tying itself in knots. I frequently passed thick blood clots, and the immense urethral burning that plagued me with this condition felt as though someone had filled my urethra with petrol and set it on fire. I often awoke at night screaming with pain because the pain of leaking urine in my sleep was so terrifying that I often thought I was being attacked.

"[The clinic] diagnosed me with a chronic UTI via microscopy on a fresh, unspun urine sample and immediately placed me on an extended course of antibiotics. Although my progress has been slow as a result of so many years of inadequate treatment resulting in a deeply embedded infection, I have finally reached the stage where my symptoms are under control and I do not require the care of urologists or my GP with regards to my bladder symptoms. I am now able to live a relatively normal life with minimal bladder symptoms, and I have returned to work and university. However, as a result of the extensive strain that my untreated chronic UTI has placed on my autonomic nervous system over the past 16 years, I have been diagnosed with postural orthostatic tachycardia syndrome, inappropriate sinus tachycardia and gastrointestinal motility problems, thought to be due to gastroparesis, which are likely to be ongoing issues throughout my life.

"My greatest regret is that so many opportunities were missed to treat my symptoms when I was a child. Had I been given early access to treatment, my lifelong suffering could have been entirely preventable. I can only hope that in the future, children like myself will not be confined to the suffering and trauma that I have experienced."

It is right to permit a parent to provide a comment and one such is recorded below.

A parent writes:

"Emma could not be potty trained and my mother, who is a retired midwife, noticed that Emma's urine smelt strongly suggesting an infection. I went to the GP several times and was told:

'The dipstick test showed no infection or not enough white cells for an infection.

The culture test came back as mixed, demonstrating a contaminated sample.'

"We were referred to the Community Nursing Team who thought Emma was choosing not to go to the toilet and we followed a behavioural program for 3 months which made no difference. We went back to the GP who referred Emma to a paediatric urologist at the ***** Hospital. The urologist had scans on kidneys and stomach completed which showed constipation. The urologist stated he did not believe Emma had a urine infection, and said symptoms described were caused by constipation. We were referred and treated for constipation by the paediatric consultant at ***** Hospital.

"I took Emma back to the GP as Emma's nursery, my mother and myself had concerns that a urine infection was being missed. My work patterns changed and I saw a different GP who prescribed antibiotics at once after a dipstick test. I returned to the GP when the infection came back a few weeks later and different antibiotics were prescribed. This went on until I had the next hospital appointment where upon the consultant prescribed a low dose of antibiotics (2.5ml cefalexin). Emma's physical symptoms disappeared and at the next hospital appointment the consultant stated he thought the infection had been caused by constipation. As the constipation was under control, and preventative steps were being taken (wiping, showers rather than baths, etc) we could take Emma off the antibiotics. The consultant had scans of kidneys and a nuclear medicine scan completed and found no defects, scarring or reason for Emma to be suffering from infections.

"While waiting for the next hospital appointment Emma suffered physical symptoms of urine infections. This was distressing and she had to have time off school and I had to take time off work. Only one GP would prescribe antibiotics. Other GPs stated there was no evidence of an infection. At the walk in clinic at ***** Hospital they also stated the white cells were too low for an infection and said Emma's temperature, pain and wetting were caused by a virus. However, they reluctantly prescribed antibiotics. Emma was prescribed many different short doses of antibiotics at this time. Often she would have to go a few days before any would be prescribed, due to reluctance/refusal from most medical staff. Dipstick tests and culture tests varied widely. It was upsetting for Emma as she sometimes wet herself in front of classmates, and she missed some school.

"At the next hospital appointment, the consultant prescribed a low dose of antibiotics and reiterated hygiene steps we could take. This all worked well and Emma's physical symptoms disappeared. My GP had written a letter to the consultant asking for more investigation as dipstick tests often showed white cells. The consultant told me there were no other tests to be completed and the infection was caused by constipation. At the next hospital appointment, I said I was concerned that Emma was on antibiotics for a long time — on and off for 3 years. I said I was also concerned that the infection still showed on dipstick tests and that Emma did not have constipation any longer. I was told she may grow out of the urine infections and that some women happened to be sensitive to infections at certain points of life.

"The last hospital appointment was a couple of weeks ago via the phone. I had taken Emma off antibiotics and the infection had come back. The culture test grew *E. coli* and the consultant suggested a short course of antibiotics followed by a low dose of cefalexin. It was suggested that I stop the antibiotics every 6 months and to restart if Emma got an infection. The consultant told me we could rule out constipation as a cause and Emma may just be sensitive to getting infections. He thinks she will 'grow out' of it in the end. I have asked if he will share care with a private urologist specialising in embedded UTIs. The consultant has refused as he has 'never even heard of embedded UTIs' and that children's anatomies are 'completely different to adults'."

CUTIC for kids is a self-help organisation set up by parents of affected children (www.facebook.com/groups/1439446326088527). We asked one of the founders if she would be willing to contribute a statement to this chapter and this we reproduce below:

"There are increasing numbers of desperate parents contacting CUTIC requesting the names of UK-based paediatricians who can treat their children for suspected embedded UTI and chronic infection. They tell us of similar medical histories, uncomplicated UTIs treated with a short course of antibiotics, only for the infection to return within days or weeks. Then, further short courses of antibiotics with infection-free days becoming less and less until symptoms become chronic. Further, parents tell of children being denied antibiotics, based on insensitive tests (dipsticks and cultures) despite having all the clinical symptoms of UTI, including a high temperature.

"Parents explain their children have been given various diagnoses including: painful bladder syndrome, recurrent UTI, chronic UTI and antibiotic-resistant infections. By the time they contact CUTIC, the children have already been seen by multiple specialists with little success. The diagnostic tests and treatments their children have been given, by secondary and tertiary care specialists, include: cystoscopy, urodynamics, bladder and urethral stretches, antimuscarinics, self-catheterisation and opioid analgesics. These interventions provide limited symptom relief [7], offer no cure [7], have significant side effects and the potential for harm [8, 9], and have been untested on children [10].

"These children live in constant pain, are unable to sleep at night, miss large parts of their education, often unable to move far from a toilet due to frequency, feel constantly unwell, and are unable to play and participate in activities with their peers. The physical and psychological impacts of the condition are devastating. It is a childhood lost.

"Unfortunately, there is little that we can offer to these desperate parents and children, as there is not a single paediatrician in the UK offering curative treatment for chronic UTI. There are several specialist centres for adults, whose consultants have offered to help the children in collaboration with a paediatrician. However, despite numerous requests from parents asking their child's paediatrician to contact these centres, they have all declined. Those parents who have the resources are now consulting with specialists in the USA to access treatment; others, without funds, have realised there is a real possibility their children will have to wait for treatment until they reach an age where they can access the adult services.

"The paediatricians have failed to acknowledge chronic embedded UTI; most are even unaware of the failings of the current tests (as are the GPs). They say their treatments are guided by the NICE guidelines, but there are no guidelines for chronic UTI. These children are repeatedly forced into guidelines for acute and recurrent UTI, and are repeatedly failed by them. There are no evidence-based guidelines on what should be done for children who fail to respond to established treatments. It does feel that the clinicians are hiding behind guidelines to prevent them from taking any responsibility to offer curative treatment for these children."

The last word...

"Without reflection, we go blindly on our way, creating more unintended consequences, and failing to achieve anything useful."

Margaret J. Wheatley (born 1944), Associate Professor of Management at the Marriott School of Management, Brigham Young University, and Cambridge College, Massachusetts, USA.

References

1. Swamy S, Kupelian AS, Khasriya R, *et al*. Cross-over data supporting long-term antibiotic treatment in patients with painful lower urinary tract symptoms, pyuria and negative urinalysis. *Int Urogynecol J* 2019; 30(3): 409-14

2. Tullus K. Low urinary bacterial counts: do they count? *Pediatr Nephrol* 2016; 31(2): 171-4.

3. Leigh Day. London Trust reverses decision to shut LUTS clinic, 20th November 2015. Available at: https://www.leighday.co.uk/News/2015/November-2015/London-Trust-reverses-decision-to-shut-LUTS-clinic.

4. Boseley S, Devlin H. In pain all the time: will there ever be a cure for chronic, life-changing UTIs? *The Guardian* (Health), 20th February 2019. Available at: https://www.theguardian.com/society/2019/feb/20/in-pain-all-the-time-will-there-ever-be-relief-for-women-with-chronic-life-changing-utis.

5. Chronic urinary tract infections. House of Commons of the UK Parliament — Hansard, 28th October 2016; Volume 616, Column 620. Available at: https://hansard.parliament.uk/Commons/2016-10-28/debates/ED698119-52F3-4B8B-8B4B-5EDE7106FBE1/Chronic UrinaryTractInfections.

6. Heimans J, Timms H. *New power: why outsiders are winning, institutions are failing, and how the rest of us can keep up in the age of mass participation*. London: Macmillan; 2018.

7. Kavvadias T, Baessler K, Schuessler B. Pelvic pain in urogynecology. Part II: treatment options in patients with lower urinary tract symptoms. *Int Urogynecol J* 2012; 23(5): 553-61.

8. Santucci RA, Payne CK, Anger JT, Saigal CS; Urologic Diseases in America Project. Office dilation of the female urethra: a quality of care problem in the field of urology [published correction appears in *J Urol* 2009; 181(5): 2390. Anger JT]. *J Urol* 2008; 180(5): 2068-75.

9. Nalamachu S. An overview of pain management: the clinical efficacy and value of treatment. *Am J Manag Care* 2013; 19(14 Suppl): s261-6.

10. ICA (Interstitial Cystitis Association). Available at: https://https://www.ichelp.org/about-ic/children-ic/#:~:text=The%20symptoms%20of%20IC%20in,had%20urinary%20problems%20as%20children.

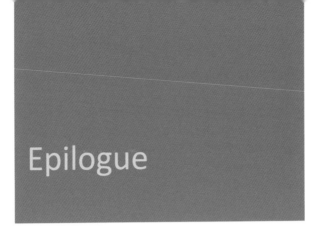

Epilogue

The *Naked Civil Servant* was a wonderful television film based on the autobiographic book of the same name by the late Quentin Crisp. John Hurt played the hero in a mesmerising performance that won him a BAFTA award for Best Actor in 1976. Quentin Crisp was a gifted, intelligent writer, but more importantly an inspiring, courageous man. He came out as demonstrably gay in the UK, pre-World War II. He dyed and styled his long hair, painted his nails, applied makeup and dressed flamboyantly; adopting extravagant mannerisms and speech to compliment these. The film is a moving tribute to the dignity of a brave human, living truthfully. At the end, a middle-aged Quentin Crisp is accosted by some duck-brained thugs in a park. They attempt to extort money from him by threatening to tell the police the falsehood that he had assaulted them sexually. In a powerful response John Hurt delivers the following lines:

"I defy you to do your worst. It can hardly be my worst. Mine has already and often happened to me. You cannot touch me now. I am one of the 'stately homos of England'."

"You cannot touch me now" has stayed much in my thoughts in the years since.

The research described through these pages occurred because our patients were unresponsive or deteriorating when we practised according to the protocols and guidelines sanctioned by the specialist groups influencing our discipline. We began to cast a critical eye on accepted wisdom and the ensuing experiments have been at the heart of this book.

What has this got to do with Quentin Crisp's assertion?

We have hinted at our adventures, and the key events have been covered in the wider press. Given the sententiousness of the comically bloated regulatory bureaucracy of our health care, it was pathetically naïve of us to believe that reporting our science and practice accordingly would ever be straightforward.

The reactions of so many senior persons to the findings we published were astonishing in their antagonism. The resourcefulness expended in efforts to stall our activities was wonderous to behold. Nevertheless, today, Quentin Crisp's aphorism "they cannot touch us now" has some purchase. The opposition seems to have run clean out of ammo. It is like the 1944 Ardennes Counteroffensive; the ordinance depot is bare.

As the smoke clears you find us standing, as merry as ever, and untraumatised by the brickbats and certainly not suffering servants [1]. We have many preposterously embellished but entertaining war stories and we can marvel at the abundance of regulatory meetings that must have happened. The research and clinical service continue to thrive. Nowadays, other centres in different nations are publishing similar results; no surprise, we did our research with such care. What on earth was all that brouhaha about? What did it achieve?

Today whilst partially retired, I remain in clinical practice and active in our research but I have stepped down from leadership. Two of my PhD graduates have been appointed consultants for the NHS service and another is head of the basic science programme at UCL. A third consultant appointment is being considered and there are six doctors serving the private practice. They follow a common protocol that was evolved as 7000 sufferers passed through our hands. There is hope, a new generation arrives, and youth will always bring change.

---

1.   Isaiah 53: 1-12.

There is a stark question that must be taken seriously now, and by all of the specialties in this field. It must cease to be an undiscussable: science has revealed serious, widespread deficiencies with errors of validity affecting all the protocols that address the management of chronic lower urinary tract symptoms. There is evidence of much consequential suffering. Reader, what will you do about it?

James Malone-Lee MD FRCP
jamesmalonelee@gmail.com

Index